Enough: When Sacrifice Has Gone Too Far

DR. ANDREA D. SULLIVAN

ANDREA D. SULLIVAN, PHD, ND, DHANP
Enough: When Sacrifice Has Gone Too Far

IMPORTANT NOTE: The Reader should bear in mind that this book is not intended to take the place of medical advise from a trained medical professional. Readers are advised to consult a physisician or other qualified health professional regarding treatment of all of thier health problems.

This book was written to provide selected information to the public concerning canventional and alternative medical treatments

Published by: Publisher House

Text Design by: Davia Lilly, Lilly Design Group

Cover Design by: Davia Lilly, Lilly Design Group

Cover Illustration: Jonathan Edwards

Table of Contents

PRAISE FOR ENOUGH

Enough explores the unique experiences of African American women and shows how too much sacrifice, often made in the name of family and racial progress, can cause profound harm to our bodies and minds. Writing with empathy, tenderness, and grace – and from a wellspring of personal and professional experience – Dr. Andrea Sullivan serves up a timely roadmap to true health and wellness. Her advice is practical, no-nonsense, science-based, and honest. It will uplift you—and change your life.

Marilyn Milloy, *former deputy editor of AARP the Magazine*

Put down your superwoman cape and read this origin story to free yourself from a life of over-sacrificing. If you pick up this book, you will not put it down, your life, your mindless habits, and real solutions are in there. Dr. Andrea Sullivan is a national treasure. She has been preaching the gospel of a naturally healthy lifestyle for over four decades. The chapters on water and sleep alone make her book a true lifesaver. I give advice for a living, but Dr. Sullivan's advice will save your life. Enough of the gimmicks, this is the remedy you need for a happy, healthy and full life.

Kim Keenan, *President of International Women's Forum of DC and Co-Chair of the Internet Innovation Alliance, Former President the National Bar Association, and the District of Columbia Bar. She is the former longest-serving General Counsel of the National Association for the Advancement of Colored People. She is putting her cape in storage.*

MORE PRAISE FOR ENOUGH

As little girls, we are told that we stand on "steely shoulders."
The shoulders of strong, faithful and courageous women who
looked out for everyone in order to survive. In Dr Andrea D
Sullivan's new book, "Enough: When Sacrifice Has Gone Too
Far," she reminds us that we have grown "sick and tired of being
sick and tired." Too many Black women are on the front lines
saving everyone but themselves. They're super-givers who neglect
themselves. Oh, they see their doctors, but they don't really get
better. Dr Sullivan believes that to save our community and our
country, we have to save ourselves.

Drawing on 34 years of practiceas a naturopathic physician,
she knows the stresses and problems that Black women face
and the health issues we must confront.

Enough is more than a self-help "practical tool kit,"
it's about charting a new narrative to save ourselves in
order to save our nation.

Donna Brazile*, Former Acting chair of Democratic National*
Committee, political strategist, FOX news political analyst,
author, syndicated columnist, and Adjunct Assistant Professor
at Georgetown University.

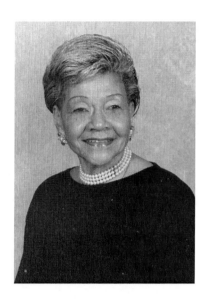

This book is dedicated to the memory of my mother
Mary Lucretia Harris Sullivan
August 22, 1919 - September 24, 2019

Enough: When Sacrifice Has Gone Too Far

DR. ANDREA D. SULLIVAN

Gratitude

The quality of being grateful, (warmly or deeply appreciative of kindness or benefits received), or thankful.

Were it not for the Grace of Spirit, and the never ending, loving and support of family and friends, this book would not exist.

Since 1986 I have been blessed to have people come to me and share their stories. They have presented among other dis-eases, their fears, secrets, shortcomings, deceptions, anger, disappointments, depression, suicidal ideations and anxiety, with the hope and end goal of healing and wellness. The women who choose me to tell their story to, honor me. I applaud their tenacity, resilience, and determination to seek something different for themselves and their families. I am humbled by their faith in me, and Naturopathic Medicine.

It's not easy to bare one's soul. It takes courage. A friend told me once " it takes great courage to see the face of God". Releasing the depression, anxiety, secrets, etc., I believe allows us to see ourselves as we truly are— made in the image of Mother/Father God/ All That Is And it takes work.

And it took much work to deliver the stories and all the information in this book. For that, I am grateful for Davia Lilly of Lilly Design. Her creativity and knowledge, humor and honest feedback were blessings throughout this process. We had difficult times through the loss of loved ones and she continued to hold the focus to completion.

I am grateful for Donna Brazile, Kim Keenan, and Marilyn Milloy, for their time and endorsements. Their successes and passions are examples for me.

Heart and Soul

Andrea D Sullivan, PhD, ND, DHANP

Behind the Cape
of a Superwoman

Answer honestly.

Are you tired of being overweight or feeling sluggish and unhealthy? Are you tired of the familiar rut of sleeping through your alarm then finally waking to a diet of coffee and donuts or some other fast-food breakfast sandwich? Are you tired of eating fast food for lunch or worse, eating no lunch at all? Are you tired of all those muscle aches, joint pain, headaches and backaches? Are you spending too much time on the couch in front of the plug-in drug called TV where you're sitting but not really relaxing? Are you tired of all the medications you have to ingest, some of which are prescribed to lessen the symptoms caused by the medications you have to ingest?

Are you tired of the negative thoughts and feelings – resentment, guilt, fear and shame – that occupy your brain day in and day out? Are you tired of being irritable, impatient, angry or anxious? Are you, in the immortal words of iconic Civil Rights activist, Fannie Lou Hamer, sick and tired of being sick and tired? And most importantly, are you tired of taking care of everybody but yourself?

I hope you answered yes to all of the above because you cannot continue to do what you have always done – take care of everyone but yourself – and expect a different result. Doing what you've always done and hoping things will change is the definition of insanity. Yet, I understand this brand of insanity. I understand that your heart is big, and you've been conditioned to be a caretaker. I understand you bear others' burdens, even though no one helps you with yours. I understand the responsibility you feel for fulfilling everyone else's needs before you take care of your own. I understand that African American women are the most stressed out and disregarded group in America (with African American men falling in line right behind us). I understand that African American women overcompensate when we don't feel good about ourselves. And I understand why we have the highest rates of chronic diseases of any group in America.

We are Superwomen.

That origin story is part of a long history. Superwoman was born out of an adaptive response to the abhorrent circumstances of slavery and Jim Crow. Superwoman sacrifices herself for others and succumbs to the "Sojourner Syndrome." Anthropologist Dr. Leith Mullings first advanced the idea of the Sojourner Syndrome in 2002 when she described Sojourner Truth as representative of African American women who resist the "interlocking oppressions of race, class and gender" that defined their existence for generations. Sojourner sacrificed herself for the good of the collective, took on numerous roles and responsibilities and, as a result endured an inordinate amount of stress that impacted her health (Mullings, 2002).[1] At age 86, Sojourner died from leg ulcers resulting from untreated diabetes.

Allow me to introduce three modern-day Superwomen, Diane, Darlene and Mary.

Diane, an African American woman in her late 30s, came to me complaining of constipation, thyroid problems, joint pain, and high blood pressure. She was a pleasant, kind woman who was short in stature and carried more weight than she wanted. She had a muscular thick in body type. Diane was stressed out from raising her grandson, working a demanding federal government job, and dealing with the emotional blow of being passed over for promotion by a young White man whom she had trained.

As I probed a little deeper into Diane's background, she recounted what she termed a "normal" childhood: her father was abusive and an alcoholic, her mother was abused, and her brother, who committed suicide, was verbally abusive. To escape the pain of her upbringing, Diane married young and gave birth to a daughter who became a teenaged mother. After marrying, Diane soon discovered her husband was being unfaithful to her. While she was going through the storm of a painful divorce, Diane's father died suddenly from a heart attack. If that wasn't bad enough, Diane's mother blamed her for the anguish and stress her father suffered, and the two of them remained estranged for years.

Darlene was a retired mother and grandmother in her late 60s when she came to see me. She was taking seventeen different medications. She had prescriptions for diabetes, hypertension, and elevated cholesterol levels to name a few. She was of medium height and weight with a sadness that surrounded her as she entered my office. Through tears, she told me about her depression. It began when her husband left her to marry another woman with three children, she told me. She said her husband was mean, violent, and verbally abusive, even after he left. She sought refuge in another relationship, but that soon ended. Darlene had raised her two children and a nephew— the son of her sister who had passed on. Now, just when she felt she should have been sitting back and enjoying her golden years, she became saddled with the burden of raising three of her grandchildren.

Mary, also retired, came to me after being diagnosed with fibromyalgia, high cholesterol, hyperthyroidism, depression, and insomnia. After she went through a nasty divorce and subsequently had to raise her three children alone, Mary never slept well. Mary found out during her divorce proceedings that her husband, a drug addict with erratic behavior, had fathered other children while they were married. While he was not physically abusive to her, she never felt safe with him— or supported.

"My husband was always off chasing other women. So many things were coming at me. I was overwhelmed, anxious, and feeling I had no control. Even now I am doing so much for others and not for myself," she said. "I make sure others are well but not me. They cannot find out what is really wrong with me. I am raising my six-year-old granddaughter because my daughter is on drugs, and I take care of my 94-year-old mother. There is always so much to do and so little time to do it. I have fears about my health and having enough money. I feel backed into a corner and afraid I cannot get things done. I just feel things are out of control."

My patient's stories remind me of a time when I was weighed down by my own Superwoman cape. At twenty-six, I earned a PhD in Sociology and Criminology from the University of Pennsylvania. I then taught graduate and undergraduate students at Howard University. When I was twenty-nine, I was working as a Special Assistant for Urban Policy for Dr. Patricia Roberts Harris, the first African American woman to be appointed a Presidential cabinet member. My typical workday went non-stop from eight in the morning until six or seven at night. Pretty soon, I was burnt out, and I knew I needed help.

I turned to Dr. James L. D'Adamo desperate to lose the weight, the chronic fatigue and the terrible acne that had been plaguing me. During my first visit to Dr. D'Adamo, a naturopathic physician, I became aware that much of my "dis-ease" had to do with the experiences I had endured growing up as an African American woman where everything from the bread to the milk to models on TV were white. As we began peeling back the layers of my past, namely sexual molestation by a neighbor across the street and the low self-esteem that followed, I shared with him that despite earning good grades in high school, my guidance counselor told me I should become a domestic worker. I told him about the shame and humiliation I felt upon hearing that and the shame that overwhelmed me when my White high school friends hid me in the basement as soon as their parents came home. I also told him about the shame I felt around being bi-sexual. Always wanting to compensate for my perceived inadequacies and sense of inferiority, I had worn myself out.

The stress that results from racism, classism, sexism— any "ism" you can name often promotes low self-esteem, negative thought patterns, and poor nutritional habits, all of which provide a fertile ground for dis-ease to develop. Additionally, African Americans contend with the everyday challenges of racism from without as well as colorism from within. In our own families, many African American women are treated differently based on how light or dark our skin tone.

African American women also bear the brunt of the effects of job discrimination, single parenting, and partners and family members suffering from drug and alcohol addictions. Some of us have suffered sexual abuse at the hands of a father, brother, mother, uncle, babysitter, grandfather, or neighbor. These traumas influence how we view the world and ourselves and how we handle life's daily happenings. Years of mental, emotional, and spiritual neglect and abuse negatively affect our physical health and wellbeing.

Then, and only then, do we seek help. Far too many women come to me after they've hit their breaking point— engulfed in their Superwoman capes, addicted to fast food, wobbling on aching joints, and popping more pills than the law should allow.

It is time to declare ENOUGH!

I wrote ENOUGH!: When Sacrifice Has Gone Too Far because I want African American women to stop dying faster and younger than White women. I want women of color to stop dying from cancer at higher rates. I want African American women to eat less fried chicken, drink more water, go to sleep before midnight, and exercise for at least ten minutes a day or three times a week. I want us to stand up and have the courage to say "No!" I want us to forgive ourselves and stop judging ourselves and others. I want every woman to know who she is spiritually and to recognize she is a precious soul where God resides. If we are truly committed to beginning the healing process, we have to develop new habits, rehearse new thought patterns, and make different choices. How do we get there? We have to start with a new understanding about the value of our health.

ENOUGH! was created to save lives, decrease morbidity, and alleviate and heal dis-ease in African American women. This book will inspire you to take control of your emotional, physical and spiritual health and wellbeing. Instead of spending your money on the best clothes, cars, jewels, and handbags, this book will show you how to invest in your health and create the kind of wealth money can't buy. ENOUGH! offers a practical toolkit that helps you make yourself a priority, repair your body, and, most importantly, prevent its breakdown.

ENOUGH! will show you how to begin the practice of caring for and loving yourself. Even if you choose to continue to be a Superwoman who guides, protects, supports, nourishes, nurtures, and loves others, you can also choose to love and nourish yourself. Giving from a place of lack just won't work. We must learn to give from our own well of abundance, strength and sustenance. It's time to don a cape woven with threads of awareness and wisdom on how to cultivate robust health and well-being. Let me ask you, do you honestly think God put you here to be sick, stressed out, and forever on the verge of a breakdown? The opposite is true. You are entitled to have good health and have it more abundantly.

ENOUGH! isn't your typical, quick fix, Hollywood fad-diet book. It is a journey of discovery into the world of naturopathic medicine and your own power to heal. Naturopathic medicine may sound foreign to women of color, but it has been the key to saving my patients' lives. Indeed, naturopathic medicine has been saving lives for centuries. Naturopaths are medical professionals who treat people, not conditions. Naturopaths carefully consider a patient's physical, emotional, mental, and spiritual states of being since each serves as the root of both dis-ease and the healing of dis-ease. Naturopaths work with patients to remedy the causes, not just the outward signs of their illnesses. In doing so, naturopaths prescribe natural substances and lifestyle changes to aid in healing and overall robust health.

ENOUGH! is about using your strengths and discipline to heal and save yourself. And save yourself you must. You cannot afford to do nothing in hopes that the systems which have been oppressing you for centuries will somehow rally to save you.

ENOUGH! is designed to help you discover how to restore overall balance and wellbeing to your mind and body. Throughout ENOUGH! you will discover specific, life-saving changes that can help you manage and combat the negative effects of stress, the Sojourner Syndrome, and the Superwoman persona. Yes! We can retreat from the brink of disaster by reclaiming naturopathic medicine. I write reclaiming since our African ancestors practiced naturopathy even though they didn't call it naturopathy.

ENOUGH! will assist you along your path to robust health and wellness by suggesting necessary lifestyle changes. On the pages that follow, I will teach you about proper nutrition and the personal growth and the stress-reduction techniques that changed my life and the lives of many others. I will also address the unique experiences in African American communities that have given rise to behavioral adaptions that negatively impact our health.

You can do this. Think about it: African Americans survived the Middle Passage, slavery, the Black Codes, Jim Crow segregation, the war on drugs and today we're battling the New Jim Crow. If we can survive those oppressions, surely we can change our negative thinking and our less than optimal eating habits.

The truth is, we can do anything. Many have led the way: Harriet Tubman, Fannie Lou Hammer, Dr. Anna Julia Cooper, Rosa Parks, Coretta Scott King and Betty Shabazz. So, if you're still thinking you're too busy saving everyone to devote time and attention to your own physical, emotional and spiritual needs, then how about this: if you won't do it for yourself, then do it for your great grandmother, your grandmother, your children or grandchildren. Better yet, JUST DO IT— for you.

It's time to say ENOUGH! ENOUGH of the sedentary lifestyle, watching TV, and snacking. ENOUGH of eating poorly and being in a state of chronic fatigue. ENOUGH struggling with your weight and ENOUGH putting off exercising regularly. ENOUGH of the gossip, negative self-talk, not loving yourself, and not recognizing that you are your greatest asset. ENOUGH of saying "Yes" all the time and doing for everyone except yourself. ENOUGH with thinking it is better to give than to receive since giving and receiving are part of the same cycle of abundance. ENOUGH dimming your light so others can shine. ENOUGH denying your worthiness. ENOUGH of the guilt, anger, resentment, and shame you carry. ENOUGH of the dis-eases, and medications. It's time to say ENOUGH!

SACRIFICE – the offering of animal, plant or human life or of some object to a deity, as in propitiation of homage; the person, animal or thing so offered; the surrender or destruction of something valued for the sake of something having a higher or more pressing claim; something so surrendered or lost;

Synonyms – loss, deprivation, privation, forfeit, expense, cost, damage, destruction, ruin...

DR. ANDREA D. SULLIVAN

CHAPTER 1

HOW DID WE GET HERE?

*"Not asking for help is an issue. I could appear vulnerable. Being
hurt is the fear...even playing Superwoman, you get hurt."*
—*Diane*

SOJOURNER TRUTH – SISTA WARRIOR

Sojourner Truth, whose given name was Isabella Baumfree, was born
enslaved in New York State around 1787. Her father was captured in Ghana,
West Africa and her mother in Guinea and they were sold into slavery.
Sojourner was separated from her family at a young age and raised under
oppressive conditions. Sojourner witnessed the sale of her brothers and
sisters and later her son. Sojourner was no stranger to heartache.

She was sold for the first time at age nine for one-hundred dollars
and a flock of sheep after her enslaver died. Sojourner labored for three

other enslavers and was often abused physically, sexually and of course, emotionally. She had three other enslavers after that, and she continued to be physically, emotionally and sexually abused. She was ultimately forced to marry an enslaved man who she did not love. She gave birth to a son James, who died in childhood, another son Peter, and three daughters—Sophia, Elizabeth and Diana. Diana was conceived when Sojourner was raped by one of her enslavers.

Sojourner ran away in 1827, the year before New York's law abolishing slavery took effect. She took only her infant daughter Sophia and escaped to a nearby abolitionist family. That family paid twenty dollars to secure her freedom and later helped her win a lawsuit seeking the return of Peter, her five-year-old. Peter had been illegally sold into slavery in Alabama (Michals, 2015). After Peter's disappearance from the ship where he worked, Sojourner felt she was called by God to travel or sojourn and speak the truth. Consequently, she changed her name to Sojourner Truth, and she became an abolitionist speaker.

While on one abolitionist tour, Sojourner attended the Ohio Women's Rights convention. Her famous spontaneous speech at the convention in 1851, "Ain't I A Woman," spoke to the oppression and resilience of African American women and the contrasting deferential treatment accorded to wealthy white women.[2]

Women were perceived as the "weaker sex" and wealthy aristocratic white women in particular were to focus solely on household duties and child rearing and leave field labor to enslaved Black women. Thus, Black women suffered under the weight of racism and sexism. Enslaved Black women suffered economic exploitation, family dissolution, sexual exploitation, and of course, forced childbearing to produce a labor pool for their enslavers. Additionally, enslaved women were used as subjects in medical experiments.[3]

SEXISM, THE SOJOURNER SYNDROME AND SUPERWOMEN

The oppression from sexism was the focus of The Declaration of Sentiments, as it was called, at the first woman's rights convention in Seneca Falls, NY. The Declaration of Sentiments underscored the following concerns: married white women were legally without rights; women could not vote until 1920; married white women had no property rights; husbands had legal power over their wives and could do things like beat or imprison them with impunity; divorce and child custody favored men; colleges and universities would not accept women; and most occupations were closed to women, especially medicine and law. [4]

Women could not serve on juries until 1960 and could not work while pregnant until 1970. In the late 1800's passports were beginning to be standardized. Then, a single woman could be issued a passport in her own name, but a married woman was listed as an anonymous add-on to her husband's document. Interestingly, the U.S. passport includes 143 inspirational quotes from notable Americans, and only one belongs to a woman— African American scholar, educator, and activist, Anna J Cooper. In 1892 she wrote "The cause of freedom is not the cause of a race or a sect, a party or a class — it is the cause of humankind, the very birthright of humanity." [5]

Combine this history with the experience of slavery in North America and you get the Sojourner Syndrome— a symbolic representation that traces our current health disparities to the roles and responsibilities that have plagued African American women for centuries.

During slavery there was little external motivation to do or be anything except a slave (other than freedom of course). The fact that many enslaved people were not allowed to marry someone of their choice (as with the case of Sojourner) often led to a lack of responsibility and accountability within our communities. Even if they wanted to be the head of the household, enslaved African men had limited opportunities to do so. In his book, Slavery (1971), Stanley M. Elkins states "'Sambo', the typical plantation slave was docile but irresponsible, loyal but lazy, humble but chronically given to lying and stealing; his behavior was full of infantile silliness and his talk inflated with childish exaggeration. His relationship with his master was one of utter dependence and childlike attachment." Elkins asks the question, was Sambo real? Clearly even in the 1900's, and maybe today, this character was seen as the product of racial inheritance. And with these circumstances came the lack of a two-person household structure and the integrity of a family unit for enslaved Africans. If you were married, there was the constant threat the marriage would end with the nod of the master. Life was chaotic and unstable. Enslaved African women, if they were allowed to keep their offspring, had to be responsible for the family.

Now more and more African American women are heads of households. African American women either can't find a job or work several jobs while bearing the responsibility for the economic, social, psychological, moral, cultural and spiritual responsibilities of our families and communities. Yet within the immediate community, there's a lack of positive role models, including models for intimacy, love and conflict resolution. African American women are under consistent and persistent psychological, emotional, social and physical stress that greatly contributes to their health disparities.

Years after being denigrated as chattel slaves, African American women were depicted negatively in popular culture as "Mammy" or "Aunt Jemima." This characterization served to keep African American women inept, less than and ignorant, as well as devoted to the white family. Then of course there was the "Jezebel" persona, which arose from African American women being sexually exploited during slavery. In response to these characterizations, the reference to African American women as "Superwoman" was born to highlight the positive attributes that developed as a result of oppression and adversity. [6]

The dehumanizing experiences we've endured for generations created a legacy of independence, strength and self-determination. Our resilience and perseverance enabled us to survive socially and economically. We have learned how to protect ourselves, our families and our communities. These adaptations have led us to become Superwomen. But being a Superwoman comes at great cost. African American women who have been vigilant, strong, resilient and brave in the face of tragedy have also suffered from disproportionate health disparities and a shortened life expectancy. Even Superman had his kryptonite.

It is no secret African American women are disproportionately represented in every major chronic disease category. African American women have greater morbidity and mortality rates than white women for nearly every major illness (American Heart Journal and National Center for Health Statistics). According to the Centers for Disease Control and Prevention, 38.1 percent of all African American men over 20 are obese, and 37.6 percent of the same population are hypertensive. For women it is worse: 54.2 percent of all African American women over age twenty are obese, 80 percent are overweight, and 45.7 percent are hypertensive (as compared to 28 percent white women in the same category).

It's time to invest in lifestyle changes that decrease morbidity and disease. It's true, many women do not know what to do to create healthy habits. Others do know, yet they continue to make poor choices. Instead of spending money on things that support us in leading healthier balanced lives, some of us buy the best clothing, cars, jewelry, nails, hair, handbags and tattoos. Retail therapy is not, in and of itself, bad, but if you don't prioritize your health, all you're left with are some very expensive handbags to go along with your hypertension.

I grew up at a time when there was talk of revolution. Though what was being said about racism and discrimination was true, I was not willing to hurt anyone because of the color of their skin or opposing beliefs. For me, violence was never an option. Now we commit acts of violence toward ourselves and each other regularly. With every indiscretion in thought, word, or deed, with every poor dietary choice, we are slowly but surely shortening our time on this planet and inviting suffering. It's time to begin the health and wellness revolution. We must be revolutionary in our thinking, speaking, vision and behavior. We must empower ourselves. We must take care of ourselves by creating healthier lifestyles for our minds, bodies, and souls. The revolution must begin within each of us, and it must begin now.

Below are the revolutionary words that will propel us forward.
Ready? State boldly:

I AM LOVED   I AM WELL   I AM GOD'S CHILD

CHAPTER 2

CONSIDER THIS

"Black women will do anything for people they love but not for themselves. 'Some other time' never comes."

—*Darlene*

The Hard, Cold Facts – The Results of Being A Superwoman

For too long I have heard many of my patients echo Darlene— almost verbatim. What they are admitting to is that they sacrifice themselves daily. They're stating that the needs and desires of everyone in their inner circle come before their own. Every day, Black women attempt to give of themselves, not from an overflow but from lack— a lack of time, energy, or money. The consequences of this are not pretty. Take a look at these statistics:

- 56.7 percent of African American women over the age of twenty have hypertension as compared to only 36.7 percent of white women and 36.8 percent of Hispanic women in the same age bracket.[7]

- While more white women are likely to have breast cancer, we have a higher mortality rate - an average of five African American women die from breast cancer every day. [8]
- Four out of five African American women are overweight or obese.
- African American women die at a 50 percent higher death rate from diabetes as White women[9].
- African American women have higher rates of HPV, human papillomavirus and cervical cancer, with mortality rates double those of white women[10]
- Only 35 percent of African American lesbian and bisexual women have had a mammogram in the past two years, compared to 60 percent of white lesbian and bisexual women[11]
- African American women have greater mortality than Caucasian women from CAD(Coronary Artery Disease), hypertension, stroke, and CHF. (Congestive Heart Failure) The mortality rate from CAD is 69% higher in black women than in white women. Mortality for black females from hypertension is 352% higher than for white females. Age-adjusted stroke death rates are 54% higher in African American than in Caucasian women, Incidence, prevalence, and morbidity figures for CAD, hypertension, stroke, and CHF are all higher for African American females than for Caucasian females.[12]

The COVID-19 crisis has shone a spotlight on the health disparities that have existed in African Americans communities for centuries. African Americans are disproportionately represented in the cases of and deaths from COVID-19. In states where Black communities make up a small portion of the population, nearly half of all deaths are members of that community. And in larger cities like Chicago where the population is 30 percent Black, we are half of the cases and 70 percent of those who died. In Louisiana, 70 percent of those who died are Black, while making up only one-third of the population. Having asthma increases one's risk of getting COVID-19 and related complications. African Americans were already three times more likely to die from asthma related causes. African American women were 20 percent more likely to have asthma in 2015. (US Department of Health and Human Services, Office of minority Health), because 75 percent of the black population live in areas that border a factory or refinery (Clean Air task Force Report, NAACP 2017). According to the Asthma and Allergy Foundation of America, African American women have the highest rates of death due to asthma.

These circumstances are directly related in part to African American women being in service positions that do not allow for tele-working (we make up 30 percent of the workforce that are caregivers outside the home), utilizing public transportation, living in poor housing and neighborhoods with toxicity in the air and water, no access to quality health care, and of course the aforementioned pre-existing health issues. And though taking care of our immune systems is more important now than ever before, the economic conditions in African American communities function to worsen our health challenges:

- US Bureau of Labor Statistics reported the unemployment rate for African American women over twenty years of age is twice that of white men and since December 2020 our unemployment rate is 8.4% compared to white women, at 5.7 %. The number of white women in the labor force grew by 263,000 in December , but the number of Black women fell by 153,00. and we are paid sixty-two cents on the dollar. White women are paid seventy-nine cents on the dollar.[13] .[14]

- The poverty rate for all African Americans in the District of Columbia, in 2018 was 27 percent. African American families with children under eighteen headed by a single mother have the highest rate of poverty at 46 percent (nationwide) as compared to only 8.4 percent of families headed by married African American couples.

- African American families with children under eighteen headed by a single mother have the highest rate of poverty at 46 percent (nationwide) as compared to only 8.4 percent of families headed by married African American couples.

- (Thirty percent of African American women work in service positions compared to 17 percent of white a women. Black women's labor market history reveals deep-seated race and gender discrimination. (n.d.). Retrieved from https://www.epi.org/blog/ black-womens-labor-market-history-reveals-deep-seated-race-and-gender-discrimination/ And almost 19 percent of African American women lost their jobs between February and April 2020 at the onset of the pandemic. Now 80% of us are primary bread winners and are heads of household.

- African American women experience poverty at higher rates than African American men and women from all other ethnic groups except Native American women; a quarter of black women in U.S. live in poverty. Black women are 3.6 times more likely as white women to be single heads of households with children under eighteen.[15]

The societal challenges enumerated above keep African American women locked in a vicious cycle. When a single mother is struggling with poverty, she may not have the time or money to plan wholesome meals for her family. Easy accessibility to refined, high-fat food makes quick on-the-go meals the solution to feeding her family. Exercise may not even be a consideration with her full schedule.

Thus, too many women are following in the footsteps of Sojourner, someone who can seemingly do it all but sacrifices herself for the collective good. Sojourner's resiliency and strength in the face of the most inhumane circumstances were heroic, and she deserves praise. But when an entire nation of women tries to take on that burden, giving more than we have and running up a debt on our emotional, physical, and spiritual resources, we pay a terrible price.

Is It Really "Soul" Food?

As a society, Americans do not value health nor recognize the impact poor health has on their lives. What else would we expect after being at the mercy of a society and a culture that promotes eating chemically laden substances and calling it food? For so long, Americans have been fooled into thinking that just because it tastes good, it's good for you. Many have actually been indulging in the opposite of what Random House dictionary defines as food, which is "any nourishing substance, eaten, drunk, or otherwise taken into the body to sustain life, provide energy, and promote growth." That definition certainly doesn't sound like the Standard American Diet (SAD).

And while it has become trendy to "eat well" or "buy organic," eating better isn't pocket-friendly for many Americans. The average consumer has to pay more for food that is chemical free, pesticide free, and actually good for you. Despite this new awareness of clean eating and eco-friendly, organic cooking many African Americans are still indulging in diets that we affectionately call "Soul Food." Soul food has its origins in slavery when enslaved people were given scraps from their enslavers table, scraps including pork, dark meat chicken, and saturated oils, that today lead to multiple illnesses. It's soul food alright. This food may provide warm feelings and memories of home, but it may take you to your home-going service faster than you anticipated.

Are We Sacrificing Good Looks for Well-Being?

Health has not traditionally been a top priority for African American women. There are many reasons for this: distrust of medical doctors, lack of financial resources and sick care delivery systems, putting ourselves last, and not making healthcare a priority. However, we live in communities where our fuller bosoms and curvier hips are celebrated. White Americans and African Americans have almost opposite perspectives about what is acceptable regarding weight. Anorexia and bulimia continue to be huge problems, particularly for White female teens, while in African American culture, it is acceptable to be heavier and endowed with larger buttocks.

Historically and currently in South Africa, having more weight has been viewed as something positive. There is a dignity and respect associated with weight that represents good health and a good life. Maasai men in central Africa have " fattening periods" to be more attractive to the women. It is thought that heavier bodies protect against wasting and illness. In many African cultures today, when a person is thin, it is assumed they are going through a difficult time, a severe illness, drug addiction, or even battling HIV.

While our African brothers and sisters have packed on the pounds with traditional yams, cassava plants, and rice, we in America think we can do the same with yams that are smothered with marshmallows or greens that have been cooked beyond their nutritional value or soaked with ham hocks and turkey necks. While most of our African counterparts are walking for miles each day, the most exercise many African Americans get is walking from the front door to our cars. Our curves are indeed beautiful, but we can't sacrifice our wellbeing for shapely curves.

Choosing Style Over Health

Our perceived lack of purposeful contributions, whether from evaluations from our bosses or partners, unfulfilled relationships and dreams, the need for instant gratification, and of advertisers encouraging food addictions, keep us romanticizing desired clothing, shoes and material things more than good health.

A potential patient told me that she could not afford to eat well, but she regularly spends upwards of $300 per month to color her hair and maintain her weave. Her monthly "looking good" budget also includes funds for pedicures and manicures, shopping sprees at Nordstrom, and weekly gambling at the local casino. Several of my patients have canceled appointments with me, they said, because they'd spent too much money with Amazon.

I'm not here to judge anyone's choices. We all have different priorities when it comes to evaluating what's most important in our lives. ENOUGH! is here to be your resource and your toolkit for creating change. New habits, new thought patterns, and new choices must be made in order to heal your wounds and move forward.

Begin this journey by starting from where you are— right now. Accept the past and be grateful for today. From this place of acceptance and gratitude, I will show you how to take baby steps toward life-saving changes so that you're LIVING a life toward wellness EVERY DAY.

Say this out loud:

I AM LOVED

I AM WELL

I AM GOD'S CHILD

CHAPTER 3

The Diaries
of Superwomen

"We black women think we can fix everything"

—Mary

Can naturopathic methods be the key to restoring your well-being and peace of mind? Let's take a closer look at how Diane, Darlene, and Mary took on their health and ultimately took back their lives.

Diane: The Stressed Out Superwoman

Diane, a thirty-something, divorced mother and grandmother, is a loner who is easily offended. She is very moody and broods a lot when she is stressed out. Although she doesn't have many friends, she is very loyal, responsible and dependable. However, because of her past experiences, she fears relying on someone and being totally committed. After one of our sessions, she realized how her stress and health problems stemmed from being generous to everyone but herself. She said, "I don't give myself the freedom to do what I should do for myself. I wait to see what everyone else is doing and then I do for myself. I am held back and want to take flight. I have to get rid of this Superwoman complex."

After discussing her symptoms and background, I gave Diane a homeopathic remedy, Natrum muriaticum, which can help patients suffering from moodiness, irritability and feelings of isolation. I also advised her to record her eating and sleeping patterns and symptoms. During the next visit, Diane commented that she felt less moody and more energetic, and she wasn't as easily offended. After recording her diet, sleep patterns, and mood for the five days, she began a detoxification diet and received colon hydrotherapy. The detoxification diet excluded processed foods, white sugar, rice and bread, and included whole grains and fresh vegetables. She ate fish twice but no red meat. She began exercising regularly and practicing yoga.

By using naturopathic medicine, I was able to treat Diane as a whole person. Naturopathic practitioners treat the underlying causes of illness, not just the symptoms. A conventional, or allopathic doctor, likely would have prescribed a combination of thyroid, blood pressure, and joint pain medications for Diane. A naturopathic approach, using homeopathic medicine and herbal supplements (e.g., I used a combination of garlic, rauwolfia, and cordyceps for her blood pressure), helped Diane's body heal itself by removing the barriers to good health. Ultimately, Diane learned how to better respond to familial stress, work stress, and she changed her poor diet and sleep habits. She and I worked together for two years, and she counted me as one of her primary care physicians. Once Diane was feeling better and had lowered her blood pressure, she began making better decisions on her own.

Darlene: The Exhausted Superwoman

Darlene, a fifty-something early retiree, came to me with, headaches, insomnia, and depression and diabetes, a condition that afflicted many of her family members. Like many of my patients, Darlene, thought getting diabetes was inevitable so she ate lots of sweets, pastries, and candy and, ultimately, fulfilled her own prophecy. Darlene was a caretaker for her father as he recovered from a stroke. She also served as a caretaker for her brother. When they both passed on, she began to take care of her mother who called on her throughout the night. Darlene turned to her comfort foods while she served as caretaker and when immediate families members passed on.

Darlene was irritable and impatient, and spent most of her time alone. She was so exhausted that she fell asleep at work. Ultimately, she had to quit working when her mother's caretakers didn't work out. Darlene felt as though her mother thought more of Darlene's siblings, who were not involved in their mother's care nor did they visit her. These same siblings criticized Darlene by saying she wasn't properly caring their mother. "I thought I was doing good, and they were saying I wasn't," Darlene told me, as she wept. "I feel guilty thinking, 'Did I do enough to help?' I just miss my father, my mother, and my family so much. It is like a hole in my heart. It is torn. I spent all my life trying to do for others, even if they didn't ask me to. I always think I will be fine. I am finding out I am not."

I helped Darlene see the connection between her diet, her depression, her feelings of inadequacy, and her loss of control. We worked together to build a nutrition plan to help manage her diabetes and found ways for her to access support without looking for comfort food or validation from her siblings. I gave Darlene salacia oblonga root, a traditional Ayurveda diabetes treatment that stabilizes blood sugar levels and improves kidney function. I also prescribed the herb berberine, which serves the same purpose. I incorporated red sage root, a traditional Chinese medicine for improving circulation; quercetin, an anti-inflammatory nutraceutical; and Ignatia amara, a homeopathic remedy that treats depression and shock from loss of loved ones. After several weeks of treatment, Darlene reported feeling less depressed. After several months of treatment, she had more stable blood sugar levels.

Mary: The Retired Superwoman

Mary, my 70-year-old patient, came to me after being diagnosed with fibromyalgia, high cholesterol, hyperthyroidism, hypertension, depression, and insomnia. Ever since her divorce and her subsequently having to raise her three children alone, Mary hadn't slept well. Mary found out during her divorce proceedings that her husband, who was a drug addict with erratic behavior, had fathered children with other women. While he was not physically abusive she never felt safe or supported.

"My husband was always off chasing other women. So many things were coming at me. I was overwhelmed, anxious, and feeling I had no control. Even now I am doing so much for others and not for myself," she said. "I make sure others are well but not me. They cannot find out what is really wrong with me. I am raising my six-year-old granddaughter because my daughter is on drugs, and I take care of my ninety four-year-old mother. There is always so much to do and so little time to do it. I have fears about my health and having enough money. I feel backed into a corner and afraid I cannot get things done. I just feel things are out of control." Mary reasoned that she had failed as a mother because of her daughter's poor choices.

I treated Mary with the homeopathic remedy, Argentum nitricum, to decrease her anxiety, insomnia, and the sensation of being out of control.

Argentum nitricum is given to people who experience the sensation of overwhelm, a pending failure, or the feeling that a catastrophe is about to strike. For Mary, these feelings began in childhood in response to the chaos brought into her home by her alcoholic father. I also prescribed the herbs turmeric and garlic, as well as flax oil, and a combination of zinc, Vitamin C , riboflavin (a B2 vitamin), amino acids and selenium. These became a part of her daily regimen along with dietary changes.

As I reflect on the diseases that plague women like Diane, Darlene, and Mary, I am acutely aware that these are not exotic, rare, mysterious ailments without treatment or understanding. These conditions are understandable, preventable, and treatable. These women were able to revamp their lives with lifestyle changes and treatments that didn't include pharmaceutical drugs.

During the past thirty-five years, I have been the vessel used to treat or prevent numerous dis-eases and conditions. Naturopathic treatment involves the use of nature and its elements to support the immune system's natural ability to heal. The treatment may include botanical or herbal medicine, nutritional or dietary changes, nutraceuticals (vitamins, minerals and enzymes), homeopathic medicine, exercise routines, and stress-reduction techniques.

All three Superwomen you read about suffered from chronic diseases caused by high stress coupled with feelings of isolation and unworthiness. In the next chapter, we'll tackle stress and how to mitigate it.

Before you turn the page, affirm for yourself:

I AM LOVED   I AM WELL   I AM GOD'S CHILD

CHAPTER 4

STRESS

*"Why do we always try to please other people, take care of
everything else, and let people walk over us? It is time to stand up."*
—*Diane*

STRESS is an underlying cause for many of our diseases. Psychological
stress is associated with heart disease, infectious diseases, and inflammatory
processes such as asthma and autoimmune diseases. Because of stress, we
are dying faster and younger, and we're suffering more. Understanding
the impact of stress and how to mitigate its effects is essential for health,
wellbeing, and longevity.

When we are stressed, the sympathetic nervous system goes into the
"fight or flight" response. When we cannot handle stress appropriately,
our bodies continue to produce stress-inducing hormones. This leads to
an increase in the production of adrenal hormones, reduced blood sugar
utilization, and decreasing insulin sensitivity, all of which is making us
more susceptible to hypertension and diabetes.

Stress also inhibits the immune system's ability to destroy foreign microorganisms and hinders white blood cell function and production. The parasympathetic nervous system, which is responsible for our bodily functions while we sleep, is also depressed during stress.

The level of stress we experience depends on how we respond to stimuli. Each of us develops different techniques to handle stress—exercise, meditation, vacations, yoga, etc. Stress can be caused by something minor, like speaking in public, or something profound, like the death of a loved one. In either instance, stress makes us more susceptible to spiritual, mental, emotional and physical dis-ease. One's susceptibility to disease changes as situations and circumstances change. Through the relatively new discipline of psycho-neuro-immunology (the study of how the mind and emotions affect the nervous and immune systems), mainstream medicine has finally acknowledged that there is a relationship between mind and body and that one may affect the other.

So, what about racism and our susceptibility to dis-ease? In A Path To Healing .. I wrote, racism is the most destructive and violent sourceof sickness and stress in America. It is woven into the historical fabric of this country, it shapes our behaviors and responses to life, and it invites stress to wreak havoc in our lives. We have all suffered from the institution of slavery. As a people, one people, our morals or standards with respect to right and wrong behavior have been reduced to a goal. Our passions—emotions and sexual desire/lust—dominate our reason and ethical principles. Just as African slaves taught their offspring, so the Caucasian masters taught theirs.

Slavery was the most demeaning act of humankind. In America, slavery was a well-designed, orchestrated system that resulted in the dehumanization and destruction of an entire ethnic group of people— in character, mind, body and spirit. Slavery created constant, obvious, immediate, and certain stress. These Africans, whose psyches were crippled, were responsible, through the generations, for our self-identity and socialization, our integrity and self-esteem. Many people of color are still shackled by the chains of the past, the products of racism and discrimination.

Poverty is stressful. Lack of education is stressful. Job discrimination is stressful. Violence is stressful. Fear, depression, distrust, and isolation only encourage poor health habits. The daily burdens of living, for many African Americans, are stressful. As Opal Palmer Adisa writes in Body and Soul: The Black Women's Guide to Physical Health and Emotional Well-Being (1994):

> Did you ever wonder why sisters look so angry? Why we walk like we've got bricks in our bags and will slash and curse you at the drop of a hat? It's because stress is hemmed into our dresses, pressed into our hair, mixed in our perfume, and painted on our fingers. Stress from the deferred dreams, the dreams not voiced; stress from always being at the bottom, from never being thought of as beautiful; stress from being a Black woman in America... (p.?)[16]

Black women have been and still are the domestic support for the nation while we are routinely negated and neglected. Black women have had to care for children, grandchildren, parents, spouses, and in-laws. Many of my patients who have already transitioned spoke of raising children they didn't know their husbands had fathered during their marriage. And so the stress continues.

All we need do is listen to the news for thirty minutes to hear about ethnic discrimination, murders of young black men and women, white nationalism, and sexual harassment by white men to understand the continuing effects of slavery.

In the wake of the murders of George Floyd , Breonna Taylor, Ahmaud Arbery, Michael Brown, Freddie Gray, Sandra Bland, (the list goes on and on) my patients ask what can we do? For starters, begin using the word "ethnicity" and stop using the word "race". We are part of a global family, we are all children of God or whatever larger consciousness in which you believe. As I wrote in my first book, we are one race – HUMAN.

Race Is Not Real

"Race" is a manmade construct. It separates and divides us. The word didn't exist until 1580 and was then used only to denote certain groupings of people sharing physical characteristics and language. By the 18th century race was used for ranking the people of English colonies; Europeans, Amerindians, and Africans. The English had a long history of separating themselves from others and determining that any people who weren't English were inferior. After failed attempts to conquer the Irish, the English turned to the Americas and its indigenous people. Subsequent wars, famine and epidemics decreased the labor supply, creating a system of indentured servants, a system that was the precursor to North American slavery.

Some of the labor in the new world was initially performed by indentured servants. Some Africans were indentured, and they worked side-by-side with whites. They worked together and rebelled together. The rebellions had to stop. It soon became obvious to the colonizers that European indentured servants were neither as strong nor as abundant as the African population. They also knew that Africans cultivated crops and had skills necessary to build a new colony. The solution was to separate the whites from the people of color.

And separate they did. The Virginia Slave Codes of 1705 was the culmination of laws passed from 1660 on and they cemented the fate of Africans in America. The code declared if a person was not Christian in their country of origin, they were considered to be a "slave." Africans, mulattos and Indian slaves were considered property. The punishment for crimes, including leaving the plantation without written permission or associating with whites, ranged from 60 lashes to having one's ears cut off to death. The law also stipulated that if an enslaver killed the person he'd enslaved while he was punishing him for a crime, the enslaver would not be criminally liable for murdering the enslaved person.

In justifying slavery, enslavers argued that Africans were inferior. It was at this time that "race" was used to sustain the inequality of Indians and Africans and continue to advance the idea of white supremacy. In 1830, a craniologist named Dr. Samuel Morton began measuring human skull sizes and determined that the skull size of white people meant they were the most intelligent race. East Asians or "Mongolians" as he called them, Southeast Asians, Native Americans and finally Africans or "Ethiopians" followed. The slave masters quickly upheld this ideology. They received further support for their racist ideology when in 1851, The Charleston Medical Journal from South Carolina, praised him for "giving to the negro his true position as an inferior race"[17, 18]

These beliefs found their way into classrooms. While studying for my PhD at the University of Pennsylvania in 1971, I had a professor of Criminology, who made the statement to our class that the size of the Negro's brain was smaller than the brain of a white person and that is why Negro's are more prone to crime and violence.

Dr. Morton, known as the father of scientific racism, made these claims before Charles Darwin's theory of evolution and before the discovery of DNA. Fortunately, a PhD student also at the University of Pennsylvania

DR. ANDREA D. SULLIVAN

in 2018, Paul Wolff Mitchell, did his doctoral work on this subject noting that Dr Morton didn't consider body size. Brain and body size correlate and are adaptations to the climate in which people live. "From an evolutionary perspective there is no reason to suppose a link between cranial size and intelligence." He further says that the racial categories Dr. Morton suggests have no biological basis.19

This sentiment was pronounced in 2000 after genetic scientists gathered samples from people who self- identified as members of different races in order to create the first complete human genome. A pioneer of DNA sequencing, Craig Venter said at a White House ceremony " the concept of race has no genetic or scientific basis."20 n 2019 the American Association of Physical Anthropologists Statement On Race and Racism was " the belief in 'races' as natural aspects of human biology and the structure of inequality (racism) that emerged from those beliefs are among the most damaging elements in the human experience, both today and in the past." March 17, 2019. (National Geographic, The Race Issue, March 2018, p. 21). In America especially, because of slavery and miscegenation we are one race – HUMAN.

Over the last few decades genetic research has revealed that all humans are closely related, we all have the same collection of genes, and with the exception of identical twins, we have slightly different versions of them. All people alive today are Africans and we all evolved from Homo sapiens in Africa. As we migrated, mutations and adaptations occurred creating changes in hair, skin color, lung capacity, blood type, etc.

So, I will say again, race is a man made construct. It separates and divides us. We are one race, one people. Division by "race" is man's will, not God's will. It was and is still used to justify and explain the need for slavery. Racism is used for justifying the continuation of a system of inequality, injustice and the accompanying self -degradation and demoralization of African Americans.

So, declare boldly:

I AM LOVED   I AM WELL   I AM GOD'S CHILD

ENOUGH!

Adequate for the want or need; sufficient for the
purpose or to satisfy desire; to express impatience
or exasperation.

Synonyms— plenty

We have been victimized sufficiently by the system, our
families and ourselves. We have been marginalized,
discounted are reduced, as was intended by the three-
fifths clause in the Constitution that labeled enslaved
African people only three-fifths of a person.

ENOUGH!

CHAPTER 5

WHAT TO DO?

*"Oh, de people never didn't' put much faith to de doctors in dem
days, mostly, dey would use de herbs in de fields for dey medicine."*
—*Josephine Bacchus, an 81-year-old ex-slave from
Marion, South Carolina*

*Colored folks was brought up on these old home remedies. Like I
tell you 'bout this fever grass hump. You know when folks in the
community—lots of 'em would make that fever grass the same day
or night and give it to >em. You know we stayed up too, with the
chillun; didn't have no doctors. These old home remedies; that's all I
ever took. Right now, you know, I ain't never been to a doctor.*
—*Mildred Graves, 84, Macon County, Alabama*

NATUROPATHIC MEDICINE

It happens all the time in my practice: African American patients, when
pondering my prescription for herbs, recount how a grandmother or aunt

or great uncle used herbal remedies. For precisely what condition of the body or spirit, or what herbs exactly, patients usually don't know or can't remember. But they remember relatives taking these natural remedies as their primary form of medicine.

This doesn't surprise me. For years I was vaguely aware of a certain "yellow bush" my grandmother told me her mother boiled and dispensed to her children for colds and influenza. But I never knew the name of this magical shrub. Was it chamomile, a medicinal herb used by ancient Egyptians and Greeks? (It is recorded that Hippocrates is the Father of Modern Medicine. However, like so much of history, the accomplishments of people of color are not included. Imhotep, a Black Egyptian was practicing and writing on the subject of medicine 2200 years before Hippocrates). Or perhaps it was hydrastis, commonly known as golden seal, which is widely recognized today as one of the most popular and effective antibacterial herbs?

Our knowledge of herbal medicine in this country is a direct, wondrous gift from African slaves and early American Indians (Lumbee and Cherokee tribes, in particular). Yet millions of Americans today remain profoundly estranged from it.

Call it folk medicine. Call them home remedies. Now, however , through more research and colleges and universities offering degrees in Naturopathic medicine, it's not simply folk medicine or home remedies. It used to be we know of it only through oral histories preserved through the ages. This is particularly true of elderly blacks living in the South. Many of them still use herbal medicine as their main source of care or as a supporting treatment. They are put off, says sociologist Wilbur Watson, Ph.D., by the impersonal treatment of the current medical system, with its endless list of doctor referrals and specialists for virtually every organ.

But the use of herbal medicine in American history is still by and large, ignored by the medical establishment. Older African Americans in the South, as well as those who have lived for decades in racially segregated neighborhoods, depend more on traditions and the wisdom of their elders than on conventional medicine. There is a belief that in rural communities, traditional medical practices should not be violated. And there are limits on how much technology will be accepted. Advancements in medical tools and techniques may complement the existing traditional system, but not replace it.

The black elderly have purposely shrouded their customs in secrecy for fear of being ridiculed or misunderstood. Similarly, when many of my patients tell other doctors they are seeing a naturopathic physician, they usually receive a snicker, dismissive gesture or a negative comment.

(For a complete discussion of the beginnings of Naturopathy in the U.S. during slavery see chapter two, "Naturopathy: The Roots " in my first book, A Path To Healing: A Guide To Wellness For Body, Mind, And Soul. Doubleday, Random House 1998.)

Some of what you are about to read is found in my first book, referenced above. I have come to understand, over the years, that learning requires repetition. Some of us need to have this information repeated again and again. We learn when we are ready to learn. Not before.

So, what is naturopathic medicine? How does it work? What can it do for you? How does it differ from conventional, or allopathic, medicine? Why does it play such a crucial role in the wellbeing of black women?

Health is freedom from spiritual, mental, emotional and physical limitations. Spiritual and mental freedom is the ability to express one's self creatively without egocentrism and to think clearly with compassion and will. Emotionally healthy people are free to experience a wide range of feelings: grief, anger, anxiety. They are able to feel these emotions and yet detach from them, maintaining an underlying sense of inner peace and balance. Not dwelling on any one emotion, they leave themselves open to the next moment, and they experience the fullness of life.

Creating good health is not the responsibility of the doctor or pharmaceutical companies as conventional medicine has led us to believe. Good health is our individual responsibility. Because of the stress of certain lifestyles, unhealthy foods and negative thought patterns, most of us are functioning below zero on a health scale of one to ten. My job is to assist people in getting back up to one using homeopathy, nutrition and herbs so they can support themselves through the rest of their healing process. The patient and I are in a partnership that involves changing his/her lifestyle. The patient does the work as well as the healing. I am simply the facilitator who believes in the body's ability to be well given the proper support.

While my medical training in the basic sciences as a naturopathic student was very similar to that of someone in allopathic medical school, my philosophy about health was and is still very different. My philosophy about health is based on principles of vitalism.

Allopathic vs. Naturopathic Philosophy

Naturopathic medicine (which is complementary medicine not alternative) is based on the philosophy of vitalism. Vitalism maintains that life is more than a complex series of chemical and physical reactions. It relies on a belief that there is a soul, that which makes us breathe, that coordinates and organizes these chemical reactions. This force allows an organism to develop, reproduce, and repair itself.

In allopathic medicine symptoms of disease are thought to be a result of a physiological reaction to bacteria or virus and symptoms are considered destructive and must be controlled or eliminated so that order can be restored. When the symptoms disappear, it is assumed that the disease has been eradicated or at least controlled.

Naturopaths believe that the symptoms of a disease are not solely the result of a bacteria or virus, but that they are the body's intelligent response to bacteria or viruses. Symptoms are indicators of the body's attempt to eradicate a harmful agent, bacteria, or virus. Symptoms reflect the innate intelligence of an organism to maintain wellness.

When drugs are given they work against the body's attempt to heal itself. There certainly are times when bacteria must be destroyed rapidly and mechanical intervention, or surgery, is necessary. However, the body needs to be supported in its effort to increase resistance and decrease susceptibility. Drugs relieve symptoms, but they don't stimulate our body's natural ability to heal. And they can produce undesirable effects. One example is the rampant use of prophylactic antibiotics for children with ear infections. Antibiotics eliminate lactobacillus acidophilus, the body's normal bacterial flora. Once eliminated, yeast is allowed to flourish in the intestines, and this causes diarrhea and nausea. Without proper support for the body, the earaches reoccur and so do the antibiotic prescriptions. This, of course, leads to an ongoing cycle.

This is not to say that naturopathy does not at times support the use of drugs in some situations. But the use of natural therapies means there is little suppression of the immune system and therefore few unintended effects. Naturopathic remedies work to strengthen and support the body's innate healing power.

Differing Perspectives of Health

Because of underlying differences in their philosophies, allopaths and naturopaths (including homeopaths), view health from different perspectives. Allopaths have a philosophy of illness. They base their understanding of sickness on the germ theory. They believe bacteria or viruses cause disease and that symptoms are the disease itself. It is not until the symptoms localize to a specific organ that allopaths classify and diagnose the disease. They usually treat the disease with drugs or surgery and measure the success of the treatment when the symptoms go away. Oftentimes, success is achieved by any means necessary, no matter how dangerous the drug.

Naturopaths, on the other hand, focus on health or wellness. Naturopaths are concerned about the health of your body and what defenses your body is using to create wellness. We are concerned about maintaining wellness not just fighting illness. We determine your wellness through conversation, by noting your emotional, spiritual, and physical well-being, and by assessing risk factors such as social and emotional stress and nutritional deficiencies. As a classical homeopathic physician, I want to know the stresses in your life, issues and challenges you have had to overcome and what effect you believe those challenges had on you body, mind and emotions. I want to know your fears, sleep patterns, and food cravings as well. For example, I may ask you why you believe you have this condition? What was occurring in your life at the time of or five years before the onset of the disease? What makes you angry or sad and what is your behavior when you are angry or sad? What is your experience of anger? Or are you impatient or irritable? Because we know that a change in one part of the body creates change in another, we must study the whole organism.

Our bodies strive to maintain homeostasis. Homeostasis is defined as the maintenance of stability and constancy while adapting to changes. Symptoms signal a disturbance, instability or an undesired change in the body. Complementary medicine practitioners appreciate symptoms because they are signs the body is creating resistance to a stressor like, for example, bacteria. A symptom is not a disease or the cause of a disease, but rather, the body's way to defend itself and keep itself well. A symptom is the best reaction your body can make when it encounters bacterial, viral, or psychological stressors. The body's only job is to keep itself well. When treating a sick patient, naturopaths attempt to stimulate the body's ability to respond to the offending agent and repair itself. Fever, for example, is a symptom all of us are familiar with. A fever is an important defense mechanism which stimulates the body's white blood cells and interferon secretions, both of which help fight infections. Eliminating the fever with a drug suppresses the body's natural defenses and prevents it from fighting off the underlying cause of the fever.

Let me offer some food for thought: have you ever gotten a headache from a lack of aspirin in your body? No. Headaches can result from a lack of sleep, constipation, dehydration, a food allergy or too much computer screen time, but never from a lack of aspirin. Similarly, do you get GERD from a lack of Zantac? Does high cholesterol occur because you haven't had enough Lipitor? In both cases, no. These conditions result from our lifestyle choices. The conventional medical establishment supports the devaluation of health and wellness via their diagnoses, caused by poor habits, stresses and lifestyle and prescribes medication to treat the problem.

Rather than attempting to control the disease or wiping out the symptom, naturopaths work to support and strengthen the body's natural healing ability and decrease susceptibility. Naturopaths refer to susceptibility as the organism's degree of strength against offending agents. Susceptibility is determined by levels of mental, emotional and physical stress.

The most recent Coronavirus pandemic more severely impacted those whose immune systems were weakened by other dis-eases like diabetes, hypertension, and heart disease and therefore, unable to respond effectively to the virus.

Lifestyle Changes

Naturopathic medicine seeks to normalize bodily functions, restore a state of wellness, and prevent disease. The philosophy of vis medicatrix naturae, the healing power of nature, is fundamental to naturopathic medicine. Using everything nature provides, I cooperate and support the body's innate ability to heal itself. As a naturopath I avoid the use of drugs and procedures that interrupt normal functioning and have unintended negative side effects. I use nontoxic therapies based on physiologic principles to treat the whole individual, not just the disease or condition, because the whole person is involved in the healing process. My concern is with the cause, treatment, and prevention of disease.

Naturopathic doctors teach patients to make lifestyle changes that focus on proper nutrition, elimination or reduced use of drugs and alcohol, stress reduction, exercise, rest, meditation, yoga and recreation. As you will read in subsequent chapters, in addition to a homeopathic remedy, my patients are given strategies for being responsible for their health, such as dietary recommendations, stress reduction techniques, and herbal and vitamin prescriptions for specific diseases. I am a primary care physician working in concert with patients to establish good health habits.

Naturopathic philosophy believes that whatever is going on inside and outside your body can minimize or maximize health. Most disease begins because of a violation of healthy living. Healthy living includes eating natural unprocessed foods, getting adequate rest and exercise, having a positive attitude, staying hydrated, living a moderately-paced lifestyle, and avoiding alcohol, drugs, and polluted environments. Benedict Lust, who brought naturopathy to the United States in 1902, wrote the following in his first editorial in the Naturopathic and Herald of Health (1902): "We plead for the renunciation of poisons from the coffee, white flour, glucose (sugar), lard and like venom of the American table to patent medicines, tobacco, liquor and other inevitable recourse of perverted appetite. We long for a time when an eight-hour day may enable every worker to stop existing long enough to live; when the spirit of universal brotherhood shall animate business and society and the church...when people may stop doing and thinking and being for others and be for themselves..." (Take care of yourself so that you can take care of others).

The scope of naturopathy is broad because we treat people, not diseases or organ systems. Every phase of life is important to the naturopath. We treat everyone from the infant to the elderly using therapies such as homeopathy, nutrition, botanicals (herbs), acupuncture, hydrotherapy, exercise, manipulation, and massage. Our specialties then are in the treatments we use and not in organ systems such as the heart, cardiology or the joints in conventional medicine since the organs are not separate from the soul.

As Lust said in 1902:

In a word, naturopathy stands for the reconciling, harmonizing and unifying of nature, humanity and God. Fundamentally therapeutic because men need healing; elementally educational because men need teaching; ultimately inspirational because men need empowering, it encompasses the realm of human progress and destiny.[21]

During the past several decades we have seen a resurgence of naturopathic medicine. I say resurgence because naturopathy is not new. Though naturopathic medicine has been around for centuries, many people, especially African Americans, have not taken full advantage of this heritage. If you haven't, it may be time to start.

HOMEOPATHIC MEDICINE

Whether an acute or chronic condition, Homeopathy considers the whole person. It is not enough to ask a person about the specifics of a headache, but we also need to know the mood and temperament of the person, their sleep patterns, anxieties and concerns (stresses) during and before the onset of an illness, food cravings, the state of their memory and concentration, and their fears, for example. I am treating a person who happens to have headaches, not the headache.

This treatment of the whole person was the result human experimentation, which was essential for Dr. Hahnemann, the founder of Homeopathy. In 1782, he was disillusioned by the practice of allopathic medicine and left his medical practice in order that he would "do no harm". At the time Quinine, which is extracted from Cinchona bark, was used to treat malaria. There was much discussion among his peers as to how Quinine was working. He took Cinchona Bark repeatedly in toxic amounts and created the symptoms of malaria. He took Cinchona Bark repeatedly in toxic amounts and created the symptoms of malaria. He then, along with his colleagues, tested many different substances from nature, by giving the substances in toxic amounts to healthy subjects, and recorded the effects. These effects reflected the curative potential of the substance because the effects of the toxicity were the same as the expressions of the dis-ease they were trying to heal. Healthy subjects were given a natural substance in high (toxic) enough concentration to disturb their well -being and stimulate their defense mechanism. The body's response (vital force/the energy of the immune system) to this foreign substance was the most intelligent response it could make at the moment, and that response was known as symptoms. The healing substance had to produce the same signs and symptoms, when given to a well person in a toxic amount. This systematic process of testing substances on healthy people is called "proving".

Being a physician, chemist and physicist, Dr. Hahnemann understood that, in order to affect the vital force (energy), a substance's energy must be compatible with that of the vital force. He knew he had to provide energy to the defense mechanism to help it maintain balance and wellness. Hahnemann used his provings to determine which substances would match the same signs and symptoms exhibited by the defense mechanism at the time of dis-ease. He had to find a way to make the concentration of the material substance non-toxic to avoid increasing the patient's illness. Finally, after much trial and error Hahnemann discovered by diluting and shaking the substance he could increase the material's intensity (energy) and make it available to the defense mechanism. A substance that was diluted and shaken had a greater therapeutic result and had virtually no toxic risk. Hence the name Homeopathy – Homeo means same and pathos means suffering; so it is to heal the suffering with something that is the same also known as the "Law of Similars".

Thankfully, Dr Hahnemann's work did not end with his death in 1843. Internationally, Homeopathy is the second most used medical system according to the World Health Organization. I've been blessed to study with some of the best homeopaths in the world. More than twenty-five years ago, I began studying with Indian homeopaths, specifically Rajan Sankaran in Mumbai India (formerly Bombay). India's use of homeopathy dates back to before 1881 when the first Homeopathic Medical College was founded in Calcutta. Now more than 100 million people use homeopathy exclusively and there are about 200,000 registered homeopaths in India.

I understood from past educational experiences and degrees that we respond to our individual perceptions of circumstances and not the events themselves. These perceptions are what we call stress. And we respond to life based on these perceptions, also known as delusions in homeopathy. We form ideas and ideologies about life and view the world through those perceptions or experiences. It is our individuality.

The stress is an experience, however, not just cause and effect. From Dr Sankaran I have learned that that experience produces a sensation that encompasses the whole person. It is not confined to the mind and body and therefore not specifically human. He writes in *The Other Song*, (Thomson Press, India 2008, p.54) "it is an experience the human shares with animals, plants, and minerals and the things that make up this earth." We each have a spirit in us as a result of some life stressors. When that spirit that we have borrowed from nature, for a survival mechanism, becomes more demanding and visible without a path for expression, it is suppressed and crystallizes as a physical, mental and emotional pathology.

Dr Sankaran states further, "... the non-human melody expressed in the human can best be heard through the language of disease. And the language of disease in a person can be heard in the way he voices his complaints, the exact sensation of his aches and pains or other complaints. It can also be seen in his perception of his situation, the words used to describe it, and the effect of the situation on him coupled with his reaction to that situation."

Though I cannot give all the information in the provings for the remedies prescribed for Diane, Darlene and Mary, I can share some of the reasons they received a particular remedy. You read in the chapter on stress how we are affected by situations we perceive as stressful. When the stress hormones are released those hormones affect our physical body and activate genes that create dis-ease.

Diane perceived and experienced her mother's displeasure of her such that she did not like her mother and was certain her mother did not like her, but rather tolerated her, especially after her father became ill. I gave her a mineral salt called, Natrum muriaticum. She believed her experience of an early pregnancy and subsequent marriage upset her parents and turned them against her. The separation from her child's father and the heartbreak she felt cemented Diane's feelings that she had to be independent and could no longer trust. These experiences presented as suppression of grief, disappointment in love, heartbreak, and betrayal. She thought often of her past and would dwell on negative experiences. She had become a loner and cried alone at home fearing it would otherwise be seen as weakness. She didn't trust anyone enough to let them into her inner world. She had very few friends and no close friends. Her physical dis-ease was a result of her immune system responding to the stress of these experiences. Had I given salt to a well person in a toxic amount I could create these feelings and sensations.

Remember Darlene? The remedy I prescribed for her is called Ignatia amara. Ignatia amara is a plant, because she had the experience of all the responses of the vital force that I know from the provings. Specifically, the irritability, impatience, sighing, wanting to be alone, having the sensation of a "hole" (void) in her heart, and the sensation the heart is torn or was ripped out after experiencing all of the deaths in her family. She also expressed guilt and was weeping during our session even though the deaths had happened more than a year ago— some more than five years ago. This was her experience of grief. All of these symptoms are energy. You cannot touch grief, guilt or a torn heart. These sensations are all energy. These symptoms are not palpable.

If I were to give a toxic, poisonous amount of the plant ignatia to a well person I could create these symptoms, even though the person had not experienced death of a loved one, or a bad break up. The toxicity could create a nervous, sensitive, moody, melancholic temperament. The remedy is not the toxic substance, but rather a diluted substance or the energy of the plant Ignatia amara. The energy of the remedy is stronger than the energy Darlene's defense mechanism created in response to the experience of grief and was able to remove the energy of the defense mechanism. Hence, "Like cures like."

Mary was given the remedy Argentum nitircum for the sensation that things were out of control. Like so many women of color Mary grew up with an alcoholic father who abused her mother. There was constant chaos and craziness in the house. She felt trapped and helpless. Mary's reaction of panic attacks, feelings of overwhelm and anxiety, as well as her physical symptoms, were a direct result of her reactions to these events. She told me that she remembers attending a school for "Colored Students" and seeing the signs pointed toward the school for "Whites Only." She said, "When we went into town we could buy from the establishment, but [we] had to go in the back door. When we went to the doctor, we had to go in the back door. It was how we grew up. I felt we didn't matter. We were the underdog. I felt worthless [and] less than..."

If I were to give a toxic amount of the mineral Argentum nitricum to a well person, the toxicity would bring about the sensations of panic, overwhelm, anxiety, helplessness, life being out of control, with not enough time to accomplish tasks, with resultant feelings of failure. There is a need to maintain order and be on tine. Physically there is an irritation of the nerves, spinal column, and mucous membranes, as well as gastrointestinal problems.

Life's experiences for these superwomen culminated in varying dis-eases or expressions of energy- symptoms. When that energy, or the false self is no longer present, they are open to create greater health and vitality; to value who they are and participate in life from that perspective. Diane had to believe she could trust again and stop dwelling on past negative experiences. Darlene's energy had to shift to knowing she did all she could do for her family and lift the guilt and grief. Mary needed to experience calm, and a knowing that things were not out of control anymore. She had not failed. She was surviving.

So, let's boldly declare:

I AM LOVED   I AM WELL   I AM GOD'S CHILD

CHAPTER 6

WHERE DO I START?

Start where you are right now, today.

NUTRITION

In A Path To Healing I have a chapter dedicated to nutrition where I include information on the detoxification diet, how to eat for better digestion and therefore elimination, and what to eat depending on your blood type. There are also sections on sugar, milk and other substances that some people call food. Twenty two years later there is more information I would like to share with you, because as I said earlier, learning requires repetition.

Before diving into those subjects let me present some information about the "food" industry. The documentary, "What the Health" offers insightful commentary on how organizations including the American

Diabetes Association, the American Cancer Society, Susan G. Komen, and the American Heart Association influence the food industry. The purpose of the documentary is to expose the inter-connectedness of some organizations and persuade people to become vegetarians. Though I do not believe that everyone should be a vegetarian, I do believe it important to understand the conflicts of interests that exist between these organizations and food manufacturers.

Companies like Dannon (maker of Dannon yogurt) and Kraft (makers of Velveeta, Oscar Mayer wieners, Lunchables) are corporate sponsors of the American Diabetes Association. The American Cancer Society takes money from Tyson chicken, one of the biggest makers of processed chicken, and Yum! Brands (Pizza Hut, KFC, Taco Bell).

Susan G. Komen, originally known as The Susan G. Komen Breast Cancer Foundation, partners with and receives money from KFC and Dietz & Watson, makers of processed meats. The American Heart Association takes hundreds of thousands of dollars from the beef industry (Texas Beef Council) and from poultry and dairy producers. It also takes in millions from fast food and processed food manufacturers.

In other words, all of these health organizations are taking money from companies that produce foodstuffs that are associated with the very diseases these organizations are supposedly fighting. The documentary makes the analogy that this would be like the American Lung Association taking money from the tobacco industry. And finally, the United States Department of Agriculture gets money from the meat and dairy industry, McDonald's, Hershey's and Dannon.

Perhaps you cannot afford all organic food and you must rely on the foods in commercial markets. Are you able to purchase one organic vegetable a week? Buy fresh kale or blueberries, things you do not peel as they are more susceptible to pesticides. Or buy a free range chicken (no hormones, tranquilizers or antibiotics) on occasion. What changes did our Superwomen make to benefit their health and save themselves?

Detoxification Diet

At the end of the first visit, I ask all my patients to record in a journal the foods they eat, how much water they drink and their bowel habits for the next five days. This exercise is not only for my benefit, but also for theirs since I've found many people do not realize how much starch or sugar and how few vegetables and fruit they eat.

Superwoman Diane began her day with coffee, bagels and cream cheese, or a sugary cereal with whole milk. Lunch was often either non-existent or some fast-food option. Dinner was usually chicken and a salad or fries. Occasionally, she would have green beans or broccoli. She snacked on chips and salsa or cashews. She had maybe one eight ounce glass of water a day and did not move her bowels regularly.

Darlene ate eggs and bacon or raisin bran with whole milk for breakfast. A salad of iceberg lettuce, tomato and tuna with onions and celery, along with crackers was her lunchtime meal most days. Fried fish or chicken salad and a green vegetable was her dinner. Sometimes she had pizza. She too snacked on chips or craisins. She drank three eight ounce glasses of water in order to take her medication.

Mary's breakfast consisted of eggs and cheese with sausage and toast for three of the five days. She had oatmeal for two days. Lunch and, at times, dinner was a processed-meat ham or turkey sandwich complimented with either iceberg lettuce or soup and crackers. Once she had white rice, beans and corn. Spinach was her only cooked vegetable, which she had with fried fish, fried chicken, or baked salmon. She consumed six, eight ounce glasses of water. She had a small bowel movement daily.

I asked my Superwomen to do a ten-day detoxification diet which was primarily vegetarian. (For a comprehensive description of the detoxification diet please see pages 69-76 in *A Path To Healing: A Guide To Wellness for Body, Mind and Soul*). Fruits, vegetables (sautéed as well as salad), raw nuts, and seeds were a major part of the detoxification diet as were beans and other high-fiber foods.

I gave each woman a list of foods that have texture and color and that were multi-grain. These foods are necessary for cleansing the system and reducing the stress certain foods put on our bodies. Fish (only the fish that swim) was allowed for two or three meals when they'd decided they just could not eat one more carrot! White sugar and rice and flour were not recommended. Since preservatives and food additives were also forbidden, my Superwomen were tasked to read food labels to make sure to avoid them. Examples of common preservatives include sodium nitrite and sodium benzoate. Some common additives are high fructose corn syrup and food colorings. I asked them to eat organic to the best of their ability. Egg whites were fine, egg yolks were not. Cow's milk was also not part of the detoxification diet.

On her next visit Diane reported she was feeling much better in every way. She said she felt lighter emotionally, happier, less moody, and that she was opening up to people and reaching out to them. She said she was not thinking as much about all the negative circumstances she had with her mother or her divorce. She also felt physically lighter because she began moving her bowels daily. And her blood pressure numbers were moving back toward the normal range.

Because Darlene had diabetes, I allowed her to have fish once daily to support her blood sugar. But I also suggested she have the fish only with vegetables, not starches, in order to have a more complete digestion and elimination. I limited her fruits and increased her vegetable consumption. If she had fruit juice it had to be diluted and all natural. She told me she was not crying as much and didn't feel depressed anymore. She said she stopped thinking about the terrible things that have happened to her. She said she told herself those things are in the past. After our meeting she said she went home and noticed all the canned foods and she read the labels. She didn't want to waste it all so she ate some of it then decided to donate the rest to a shelter.

Over time, her morning blood sugar level was closer to normal not elevated as it had been in the past. She had a day when she ate a fried chicken sandwich on white bread along with some chocolate and she immediately noticed how awful she felt. Though Darlene had been taking seventeen medications, she eventually required only two. She proudly shared with me that she'd been doing really well and "I said hello to the new me."

Mary reported that she'd begun sleeping better as her anxiety and depression "really tapered off." She said she didn't get so upset about things anymore, her fears had decreased, and she was not feeling as out of control. Additionally, her pain was reduced after and she said she felt balanced and better. "I used to put me on hold. I don't do that anymore."

Diets For Blood Types

White flour, sugar and milk are not good for anyone. However, I first learned from Dr. James L. D'Adamo, my Naturopathic physician, that real foods that were good for some people, were not good for others. (Dr James L. D'adamo, *One Man's Food Is Someone Else's Poison*. Health Thru Herbs, Inc,

1980 Toronto) (His son Dr. Peter D'Adamo. expanded his father's work in his book, *Eat Right 4 Your Type*, G.P. Putnam's Sons,1996 New York)

I was a vegetarian for 8 years when I met Dr. D'Adamo in 1978. I was tired all the time, had a face full of acne and was overweight by 30 pounds. Every year I'd get a cold and a sore throat. My blood type is B positive. Dr. D'Adamo told me I should not be vegetarian and that animal protein was important for my body because of my blood type. That awareness changed my life, my career and my health. Most of the information he taught me I have seen to be true in my practice, and I prescribe blood type diets for every patient.

After years of study in Europe, he observed that people needed different types of diets depending on their blood type. Understanding that all blood types can receive blood from blood type O's, it was thought that Blood type O's were the first blood type in our human evolution. Blood type O's were hunters and roamed their environment looking for animal protein for their nutrition. Generally speaking, people with this blood type have a highly energetic and active body. In my 34 years of practice, I have found people with this blood type need physical activity not only for their bodies, but their memory and concentration as well. While exercise may not be what they want to do, it is an absolute necessity for better health. Perhaps more than any other blood type, aerobic exercise is one of the best treatments for blood type O's. They are muscular and brawny generally and require intense, frequent exercise to stimulate themselves and their minds. Without this exercise there is a tendency to laziness and lethargy. Exercise is also important because it helps the body release toxins from the uric acid build up from animal protein that they also must eat.

In an ideal world, an O should not be vegetarian and should consume animal protein like chicken, lamb, bison, fish (not shellfish) and turkey—all free range preferably. Starches and many beans are not something the O digests easily. Meat and vegetables are ideal unless there is some cancerous process. In that case I would have them to be vegetarian for a time and then resume animal protein –only fish. They cannot get all their nutrients from foods and nutritional supplements are advised. Blood type O's are reliable and conscientious people/ employees, being willing to take on the work of others and see it through to completion. They can tend to be very methodical and do not like to be rushed.

Blood type A's came into existence as we migrated out of Africa and mutated. These mutations included changes in facial structure, skin color for the ability to absorb more Vitamin D, A's do not have high levels of hydrochloric acid that O's have and thus meat is not well digested. A's were people who didn't choose to continue to roam looking for animal protein, but rather build communities and cultivate crops. Their food requirements are of a lower vibration food, like the vegetable kingdom (a carrot has less energy than a cow or chicken). A's are very sensitive. And foods that do not agree with them can create rapid responses like headaches, or acne. Being vegetarian is ideal for an A.

While my suggestion to patients to do a detoxification diet for 10 days is fairly sudden, I do not advise a sudden switch to being vegetarian in the long term. Stop red meats first, then chicken and poultry and then fish. This may take 6 -8 months to accomplish. As I say to all my patients embarking on new habits, guilt is not an option. Do your best with each meal.

A's are the opposite of O's in that they have a low vibration body and a very active nervous/ mental system. They are busy. A's are more mental, O's more physical. Blood type A's always have a thought, plan, or project, so much so they cannot do it all. They have a lot of high nervous mental energy. Of course, all people can be impatient, and A's seem to be more impatient, and can therefore experience problems sleeping. Anxiety and worry are a big part of their lives. They function on this mental nervous energy and therefore jogging and boot camps (except for weight loss) are not recommended as they will excite and exhaust the A. Swimming, cycling and race walking are great aerobic exercises for an A. And for the mind, the softer, gentler martial arts like tai chi, aikido, and qigong (chi gung) help calm the central nervous system. While I recommend Yoga and meditation for almost everyone, A's benefit greatly from practices that calm the mind.

Blood group B combines the best of both worlds – the intellect and empathy of the blood group A and the need for physical activity of blood group O. Moderation is the key for a B, however. They need to be vegetarian three to four days a week and have animal protein (fish, turkey, lamb, rabbit) two or three days a week. The dietary requirements resemble both A and O. Like blood type O's whole wheat is too acidic for B's, and corn, buckwheat and peanuts can be problematic. To receive vegetable protein, beans are better for B's than tofu or tempeh. Unfortunately, chicken is not a food that B's assimilate well. There is a type B agglutinating factor in the muscle tissue of the chicken that causes blood to clump, causing immune disorders and strokes. Fish is the animal protein source that works well for B's, especially, halibut, sole, sardines, flounder, cod, salmon, grouper, and monkfish.

It is thought that blood group B's had to be more flexible and creative in order to survive the intermingling of cultures of the O's and A's. There was not the need for the order of the A society and yet they also did not need to be nomadic and look for meat as the O once did. Type B's are more flexible and not so intense in their body or mind. Both mind and body are cultivated equally. They see others points of view and are empathetic, making good counselors, communicators and motivators.

Blood type B's could consider self-employment as they are self starters and do not do well with management from/by others.

Types of exercise are also shared with O and A. There should be some intense exercise 3 times a week for the physical body of a B, and yet their mind and nervous system also need the calming effects of yoga and meditation.

Finally, blood type AB, or the "universal recipient", came into existence. This is a rare blood type, as only about four to five percent of the population have this type. While they are a combination in personality type of A and B, they are not as sensitive as an A and have less nervous energy. High strung like an A and yet centered or easily gravitating to centering practices like a B, they are very diplomatic and pleasant. They are stronger in personality and stamina than an A, able to tolerate moderate exercise like cycling without the nervous system being taxed. They also need calming exercises like yoga and tai-chi. Their foods are very similar to an A, and being vegetarian would be acceptable. However, they should have fish once – twice a month, and do well with lamb, as a blood type B. Unlike a B, tofu is well tolerated by blood type AB's.

Find out your blood type and explore these suggestions. Perhaps it will assist in changing your life too.

Drink More Water

Water makes up almost 70 percent of our body composition. The body is approximately 60 percent water, the brain is approximately 70 percent water and the lungs are 90 percent water. Every cell, tissue and organ has water in it. We need to drink one-half our body weight in ounces. If you are an athlete or breastfeeding, you will need more water (one liter per hour of exercise). For example, if you are 150 pounds you need to consume seventy-five ounces of fluid a day mostly by drinking pure water.

We lose water daily in our perspiration, bowel, urine, and respiration (breath), and we must replace it. Lack of water causes dehydration which reduces the amount of blood in your body forcing your heart to pump harder to deliver oxygen-bearing cells to your muscle. Thus dehydration causes faster breathing and a faster heart rate. It also causes poor sleep since it blocks the production of melatonin, a hormone from the brain which helps us sleep. Dehydration is connected to time of day, rising at night and decreasing in daytime, constipation, irritability (which can be from constipation), dizziness, headaches, poor memory and concentration, impaired judgment, fatigue (water aids in breaking down and transporting nutrients to use as energy), dry skin, decreased coordination, muscle weakness, yellow urine, and blood pressure changes, as your blood is thicker and blood flow therefore restricted.

If you are thirsty you are already dehydrated.

What About Other Liquids In Place Of Water?

It is true that you can get fluids through other sources such as herbal teas and foods that are 85 to 95 percent water like celery, cucumbers, oranges and melons. Twenty percent of your fluid needs can come from foods composed of water. However, most of your fluid intake should be from pure water.

I am often asked about black tea, coffee, soft drinks, juices and cocoa? You can make an argument for any liquid as a substitute precription drugs, there are unintended side effects. The caffeine in these liquids can be dehydrating for the body. Caffeine, found in four of the five liquids named above acts as a mild diuretic in the body, causing more urination.

But more importantly, caffeine removes calcium from the bones and that can increase the risk of osteoporosis as we get older. And of course, we know coffee can produce, anxiety, heart palpitations, digestive problems, heartburn, ulcers, constipation, diarrhea, and sleeplessness.

Decaffeinated coffee is not much better. Decaffeinated green tea would be a better option. Soft drinks can create the same effect and they also contain harmful sugar. Sodas are the number one cause of type 2 diabetes in this country. And the diet sodas are worse. They may contain aspartame, a substance that has methyl alcohol which when entering the body turns to formaldehyde. Formaldehyde is carcinogenic. When aspartame and carbohydrates are mixed it causes your brain to slow the production of serotonin. Serotonin is the hormone that allows you to feel happiness and balances your mood. Diet sodas also trigger the body to believe there is sugar in the blood and thus activate insulin from the pancreas. When there is no sugar to be found the body craves sugar. These substances also have purines (which causes a form of arthritis called gout) and other toxins. Most of the water in these substances is used to eliminate toxins out of the body. And the milk in cocoa milk is not a drink really. Milk is for baby cows. The best source of fluids is still water.

What Does Water Do For Us?

Water helps to lubricate the spinal cord and joints, as well as mucous membranes of our nose, mouth and throat, aids in digestion, and flushes toxins out of the body. If the toxins are not flushed they get stored as fat cells. Water protects the brain by delivering glucose to it and keeps the body's temperature normal. If weight loss is your goal, drink the required amount of water, as it reduces your hunger. Without adequate water the organs wrinkle and weaken, like the largest organ, the skin. Collagen is affected by dehydration and that affects the firmness of the skin.

A 2016 study from University of Illinois printed in *Journal of Human Nutrition and Dietetics* that examined the dietary habits of more than 18,300 U.S. adults found the majority of people who increased their consumption of plain water – tap water or from a cooler, drinking fountain or bottle – by one percent reduced their total daily calorie intake as well as their consumption of saturated fat, sugar, sodium and cholesterol.[22]

Water, or its lack (dehydration), can influence one's mental and emotional state. Mild levels of dehydration can produce disruptions in mood and our ability to reason and learn. This may be of special concern in the very young, very old, those in hot climates, and those engaging in vigorous exercise. Mild dehydration produces alterations in a number of important aspects of brain function such as concentration, alertness and short-term memory in children (10–12 y),[32] young adults (18–25y)[53-56] and in the oldest adults, 50–82y.[57] As with physical functioning, mild to moderate levels of dehydration can impair performance on tasks such as short-term memory, perceptual discrimination, arithmetic ability, visual-motor tracking, and psychomotor skills.[53-56]

Dehydration is a risk factor for delirium and delirium presenting as dementia in the elderly and in the very ill.[65-67] Recent work shows that dehydration is one of several predisposing factors in observed confusion in long-term care residents.67 Chronic dehydration can lead to fatigue, heartburn, arthritic pain, back pain, headaches, colitis pain, and leg pain. Good hydration is associated with a reduction in urinary tract infections, hypertension, fatal coronary heart disease, venous thrombo-embolism, and cerebral infarct and all these effects need to be confirmed by clinical trials.[23]

In 1995, Dr. F. Batmanghelidj wrote the book, *Your Body's Many Cries For Water.* Reprinted in 2006, he writes," Chronic cellular dehydration painfully kills. Its initial outward manifestations have until now been labeled as diseases of unknown origin." He further notes "...water is a natural medicine for a variety of health conditions."

Let's look at histamine. Allergies are caused by a histamine reaction in the body in the event of an allergic reaction, and hydration has an effect on histamine levels. Histamine is involved in the inflammatory response and it is our body's way of responding to foreign substances. It can be released in the nose or mouth, causing the tiny blood vessels to be more open to white blood cells (part of our immune system) that actually attack the foreign substances. This reaction causes fluid to move out of the tiny blood vessels and creates a runny nose and watery eyes. When the body becomes dehydrated, histamine levels rise to help preserve water in the body. Water regulates histamine.

It is a neurotransmitter that has two functions, immune support and water regulation. When your body is hydrated histamine is barely noticeable. When you are dehydrated histamine is reacting. It is also triggered when your internal environment is acidic and dehydrated. It is produced to begin the process of water regulation when dehydrated. And because of our SAD (Standard American Diet) many of us are acidic which causes inflammation, which triggers histamine production. The acidity and the dehydrated body keep one in an irritated inflamed state.

I suggest the following to all my patients:

START EACH DAY WITH 2 TO 3 GLASSES (8 TO 10 OUNCES) OF WATER WITH SOME FRESH SQUEEZED LEMON OR LIME.

(If you are blood type A or AB, the water needs to be warm, and if you're blood type O or B, the water should be room temperature).

IN BETWEEN BREAKFAST AND LUNCH AND LUNCH AND
DINNER DRINK 2 TO 3 MORE DEPENDING ON YOUR WEIGHT.
IF YOU HAVE ALREADY MADE THIS A HABIT, DRINK ONE
MORE GLASS OF WATER A DAY THAN NORMAL

Do this weekly until you achieve your desired goal. If it is winter it is
fine to drink warm water, but no sugar.

REDUCE SUGAR

Ketchup, barbeque sauce, soup, low fat yogurt, granola, fruit juice,
sports drinks, spaghetti sauce, chocolate milk, coffee creamers, iced tea,
protein bars, cereal bars, canned fruit, canned baked beans, breakfast
cereals, premade smoothies, soft drinks, pastries, ice cream, candies,
syrup – need I go on – all contain sugar. And not the natural sugars. That
is why I have been telling patients for years to read the labels.

What words are you looking for to let you know there is sugar in the
product? Dextrose (produced from corn), maltodextrin, maltose, fructose,
high fructose corn syrup, galactose, and sucrose. Be aware also that if any
of these words are the first or second ingredient listed on a product label,
there is a lot of sugar in the product.

Sugar is made from sugar cane or sugar beet stalks. It is cut down and
sent to a factory to extract the cane juice. Molasses is present in sugar and
it is removed with water and bone char – yes the bones of animals, that
are crushed and burned then mixed with water to take out the molasses
and create the white crystals. Brown sugar contains slightly more molasses
than refined sugar. According to PETA (People for the Ethical Treatment
of Animals), the cattle bones are from Pakistan, India, Afghanistan and
Argentina. They are sold to traders in Scotland, Egypt, and Brazil who
sell them to the US sugar industry. Turbinado sugar or "sugar in the raw"

is only boiled once and so is less refined than white sugar and bone char is not used. However, both white sugar and Turbinado sugar have the same calories and carbs.

In animal studies, sugar has been found to produce more symptoms than is required to be considered an addictive substance. Animal data have shown significant overlap between the consumption of added sugars and drug-like effects, including bingeing, craving, tolerance, withdrawal, and opioid effects. Sugar addiction seems to be dependent on the natural endogenous opioids (hormones for pain relief, increased mood and lessened anxiety) that get released upon sugar intake. In both animals and humans, the evidence in the literature shows substantial parallels and overlap between drugs of abuse and sugar, from the standpoint of brain neurochemistry (brain hormones) as well as behavior.[24]

The most important brain hormone is serotonin. It is made from tryptophan, an amino acid. It is needed for mood stabilization and happiness. Tryptophan is found in eggs, cheese, tofu, salmon, nuts and seeds, turkey, and pineapples. Exercise, positive thoughts, high fiber diets, to increase gut bacteria, and sunshine also increase your levels of Serotonin.

Beta-endorphins, another type of brain hormone, are released from the pituitary gland in the brain during stress and exercise. They act on the opiate receptors in the brain, promoting pleasure and reducing pain. They are also the reason why we crave comfort food. Fatty, sugary, highly processed foods, like cakes and pies, macaroni and cheese, potatoes and french fries all raise our blood sugar rapidly and the beta-endorphins follow. As with serotonin, exercise, meditation and sunshine increase Beta-endorphins. Herbs and foods including ginseng, oranges, grapes, strawberries and chocolate (preferably 85 percent or higher cacao, vegan, low sugar, and with no artificial flavors or preservatives), are also a great option.

Randomized clinical trials and epidemiologic studies have shown that people who consume added amounts of sugar, especially sugar – sweetened beverages, tend to gain more weight, be obese, and have type 2 diabetes mellitus. In addition, they have increased triglycerides and cholesterol that lead to clogged arteries, cardiovascular issues and hypertension. Basically, sugar leads to cellular inflammation and chronic degenerative disease.

Added sugars include all sugars used in processed or prepared foods, such as sugar-sweetened beverages, fruit drinks, dairy desserts, candy, ready-to-eat sugary processed cereals, white flour yeast breads, and white rice that turns to sugar in the body.[25]

While no form of sugar is good for you, there are sugars that are less harmful such as stevia leaf extract, Sucanat, erythritol and monk fruit. You may be wondering why I didn't mention agave nectar. Agave nectar is primarily fructose. While fructose doesn't affect blood sugar significantly, regular consumption may increase cholesterol and triglycerides, as well as increase risk of fatty liver disease and insulin resistance.[26, 27]

Stevia comes from a plant called Stevia rebaudiana and has been used for hundreds of years. It is sold as a highly concentrated liquid or in packets. Being much sweeter than table sugar, you only need a small amount. Always get the ninety-five to one-hundred percent Stevia extract, or there may be fillers and sugar alcohols in the product.

The best thing about stevia is that it is carbohydrate- and calorie- free. Studies have shown that Stevia does not increase blood sugar levels as does sugar or other artificial sweeteners. Adults who ate a 290 calorie snack made with stevia, ate the same amount of food at the next meal as those who ate a 500 calorie snack made with sugar. They also reported similar fullness and satisfaction levels. Stevia does have an aftertaste.[28]

Animal studies show an improved sensitivity to insulin, the hormone that lowers blood sugar, and the release of some appetite suppressing hormones. Other studies have linked Stevia consumption to decreased triglycerides, which are not so good fats, and increased HDL (good cholesterol) levels, creating a lesser risk of heart disease.[29]

Sucanat is a natural cane sugar that is also made by extracting the juice from the sugar cane. It is less processed and needs no chemicals or bone char to get it from a plant to consumption. It is made up of sucrose, glucose and fructose not just sucrose, like granulated sugar. It retains some molasses (which remember comes from refining sugar cane or sugar beets) and also has trace nutrients like iron, calcium, potassium and vitamin B. It is still sugar and therefore can affect your blood sugar.

Erythritol is relatively new even though it was discovered in the 1800's. It wasn't until the 1990's that Japan began to use it in their foods. Erythritol is made by fermenting the sweet, natural starches in fruits like pears and melons. Basically, good bacteria eat the starch and turn it into erythritol. It's similar to the fermentation process of yogurt, wine and beer. It does not taste as sweet as sugar, and it also doesn't cause an increase in insulin levels. Erythritol is not absorbed into your digestive system like sorbitol or xylitol, which can cause digestive problems. Some of it is a chemical compound made from the fermentation of corn. As with all sugar, use sparingly.

Monk fruit is much sweeter than table sugar, has no calories or carbohydrates and does not raise blood sugar. To date, it has no known side effects. The sweetener is derived from the dried fruit, which is a small melon native to southern China. It has been used in Traditional Chinese Medicine for decades as an anti-inflammatory agent, to reduce sore throats and upper respiratory congestion, and to keep blood sugars stable. More research is needed, however, to determine its effectiveness.

WHATEVER YOU DO AVOID ASPARTAME, SUCRALOSE AND SACCHARIN. USE ALL SUGAR IN MODERATION.

DO NOT DRINK OR EAT DAIRY

Every one of my patients will say that for years I have been telling them milk is for baby cows, not humans. Not only are we the only animal that drinks milk as adults, but we are also the only animal that drinks milk from another animal. You will never see a giraffe go to a kangaroo, or a rabbit go to a mouse for milk. Even cows do not go back to their mother's after their four stomachs are formed. They eat plants! It would be like breastfeeding at age five. Dairy products includes yogurt, Lactaid, cow's cheese and butter.

"We could be putting gorilla milk on our cereal or having zebra milk and cookies. Why cow's milk? Using the animal that produces the largest quantity of milk but is more easily housed than an elephant means more money for the farmers," say the authors of *Skinny Bitch*, Rory Freedman and Kim Barnouin. It's all about the money needed for advertising and packaging. The dairy industry is a multibillion dollar industry.

So, what's wrong with cow's milk? I'm glad you asked. Milk and other dairy products are the top sources of saturated fat that clogs arteries. Milk also contains cholesterol. Diets high in saturated fat and cholesterol increase the risk of heart disease, type 1 and type 2 diabetes, and Alzheimer's disease. Studies also have linked dairy to an increased risk of breast, ovarian, and prostate cancer. [30, 31, 32]

And countries that consume more dairy have higher rates of multiple sclerosis.[33]

We need the enzyme lactase to digest the lactose, or sugar, in milk. Between the ages of eighteen months and four years, we lose the majority of the enzyme. Most of the world's population cannot digest cow's milk because of a lactose intolerance, and milk is the most common self-reported food allergen in the world. [34]

When the undigested sugar mixes with cow's milk it creates a growth of bacteria in the intestines causing an acidic environment and subsequent inflammation— and even cancer.[35] Flatulence, gas, bloating, cramps and diarrhea can follow. Another pro-inflammatory property of milk is D-galactose, a breakdown product of lactose.

Pasteurization destroys enzymes that help break down proteins, diminishes vitamin content, and denatures the proteins in milk. Undigested milk proteins in the small intestine can damage the lining of the gut, cause inflammation, and affect the body's ability to absorb nutrients.

You may have seen A2 milk. What is A2 milk? Another way to get you to buy milk. There is some evidence that a proportion of people have an inability to digest casein, a protein found in dairy. This protein is divided into 2 types, A1 and A2. Only cows' milk in the western world contains A1, due to evolution of the protein, as cows were bred to be larger and produce more milk. All other milk including human, goat and sheep's milk contain A2 protein which is easier to digest. The A2 milk company says their milk is easier to digest. Unfortunately, the symptoms of lactose intolerance and removing A1 from milk are very similar.

As mentioned, cow's dairy is acid forming and therefore alters the pH balance of body. This results in a weakening of the bones. A study in Sweden found that women consuming more than three glasses of milk a day had almost twice the mortality (more than twenty years) compared to those women consuming less than one glass a day. And those who drank more milk did not have improved bone health, rather, they had more fractures— particularly, hip fractures.

In contrast, people living on continents like Africa and Asia who do not drink much milk have decreased rates of osteoporosis. African women do not suffer from the same rates of osteoporosis as American women. Of the forty tribes in Tanzania and Kenya, only one tribe suffers with osteoporosis – the Masai. The Masai own cattle and drink milk. Higher dairy intake has been linked to increased risk of prostate cancer.[36]

Milk intake has been implicated in acne, ear infections, frequent colds and constipation. In my practice, when I've encountered children who have frequent colds or eczema, I take them off of milk immediately. That action alone reduces the number of colds and the eczema. The homeopathic remedy and herbs I prescribe complete the job of restoring the child to good health.

"Dairy products produce mucus." There are arguments and studies for and against this statement. It depends on who is funding the study as to what results are published. I encourage you to test yourself. Stop drinking milk for ten days, then start drinking it again for ten days. You decide if it's good for you.

Eat some tofu, tempeh almonds, leafy greens (kale, collards, mustards, bok choy), okra, kelp, seaweed, broccoli, beans, and nut milks to get calcium. And for your vitamin D needs, eat more mushrooms, wild caught mackerel, herring, salmon, sardines and tuna, eggs in moderation, and get some sunshine.

Finally, during this season, all of my patients are taking Vitamin D3 2000-5000 iu's a day depending on their levels and Vitamin C 1000-3000 mg a day.

You're well on your way, so affirm for yourself:

I AM LOVED   I AM WELL   I AM GOD'S CHILD

CHAPTER 7

Sleep
(What A Concept)

Whether I ask the question how much water do you drink or how much sleep do you get, the answer is the same. "Not as much as I should." Repeatedly, my new patients tell me they are fatigued and may get five to six hours of sleep per night. Many go on to tell me that they have the TV on a timer so it turns off once they're asleep. Or they report reading, working in bed, looking at their phones, playing a video game, or checking the internet until their eyelids meet.

Your bedroom is not your office, family room or den. And if it does function as all three, you've got to create some boundaries. Your bedroom is where you go to rest, sleep and be rejuvenated. I counsel my patients to remove the TV from the bedroom and put phones, laptops, I-pads, and all electronics in another room at least one hour before getting into bed. Mental activity may increase stress hormones before bed. And the blue light from your devices blocks melatonin, the hormone needed to make us sleepy. You can install a blue light blocker or get a pair of blue light blocking glasses if it's imperative for you to use your devices before bed.

I ask all my patients to go to bed the day before they wake up. So, go to bed before midnight and wake the next day preferably after seven to eight hours of sleeping. All too often patients tell me they do get seven hours of sleep. It's just that those sever hours are from one in the morning to eight in the morning. Let's look at why this is not ideal.

There are four stages of sleep. Our brain activity begins to slow down, indicating phase one and then phase two of light sleep. This is followed, hopefully, by deep stage three and four sleep. This phase is the most difficult from which to awaken. It may not be the eight hours of sleep that people say makes them tired but rather, at which part of the cycle you wake. Without deep sleep we have a higher risk of cardio-vascular disease, diabetes, obesity, and stroke, Deep sleep promotes growth hormones, immunity, bone and muscle repair and growth, and counteracts aging. The brain processes what we learned during the day.

REM sleep begins next after ninety minutes of sleep, as we sleep in ninety-minute cycles, non REM (rapid eye movement), and REM. Non-REM (stage three and four) is deeper and more restorative.

The bulk of deep sleep should be the first one to four hours of sleep, and the final half of sleep should have the longest REM sleep, but no more than 25 percent of total sleep time or two hours. There are also more non-REM cycles in the beginning of the night. As the sun rises there is more REM sleep. This is when dreams are more readily available. Regardless of when you go to bed, the shift from non-REM to REM sleep happens at certain times. So, going to bed after midnight, means you are losing that part of sleep that is most beneficial. This is clearly a problem for night shift workers and bartenders. Shift work has been linked to heart disease, obesity and cognitive issues.

There is an area in the brain called the circadian timer which matches the movement and function of cells to the levels of light and darkness with the rotation of the earth every twenty-four hours. Several chemicals are released within a daily cycle that support the sleep-wake cycle (a circadian rhythm of sleep and wakefulness). For example, Serotonin is made as soon as your eye perceives light and tells your body it is time to wake up. Serotonin stimulates your brain waves. Adenosine is a drowsiness compound that builds up in the brain during the daytime. As darkness comes there are messages sent through the eyes to the pineal gland, and serotonin is turned into melatonin, using the essential amino acid, L-tryptophan.

Melatonin is a hormone released by the pineal gland in the evening telling us it is time to sleep. Its production is highest between two and four o'clock in the morning. The higher the stress hormones of adrenal cortisol in the body, the lower the amounts of melatonin.

The sleep-wake cycle is affected by light, temperature and food. that helps to keep us on a 24-hour schedule. So bright lights at night including our TVs and devices create wakefulness. The circadian rhythm, or internal clock, keeps the body in sync with the sun. This body clock controls not only waking and sleeping, but also body temperature (lowest before dawn), blood pressure regulation (highest in the evening), alertness (highest in mid-morning and early evening), intestinal activity (peaks in the morning), and hormone production. The ninety minutes before midnight is the time the body is most replenished and cells are restored. It is also the best time to bring the adrenaline levels down. Adrenaline is the hormone responsible for the fight or flight reaction when you are stressed.[37]

And believe it or not, your genetic makeup dictates whether you're more comfortable going to bed earlier or later within that rough eight-to-midnight window, says Dr. Allison Siebern, an insomnia and sleep expert and professor in the Stanford University School of Medicine. "That means night owls shouldn't try to force themselves to bed at nine or ten if they're not tired. Of course, your work schedule or family life may dictate when you have to get up in the morning. But if you can find a way to match your sleep schedule to your biology—and get a full eight hours of Z's—you'll be better off," she said. So, go to bed. I tell my patients just go to bed around ten or eleven, two nights a week to start and see what happens. I suggest to them:

- Have a routine (turn off all devices an hour before bed, take a shower and as the body temperature drops you should become drowsy) and a schedule;
- No alcohol, coffee, caffeinated tea or food before bed. If you have to eat, eat protein not carbohydrates
- (breads, potatoes and pastas);
- Do not drink anything before bed; or after dinner;
- Instrumental sleep music before getting into bed is fine;
- Use white or pink noise if you have to have anything;
- Avoid excessive exercise (stretching, yoga is ok);
- Use an eye mask and ear plugs, the kind for swimmers) if you are sensitive to light and noise;
- Stimulate an acupuncture point behind and below ear with your finger;
- Put the temperature on 65-68 or whatever is cool to them, as this makes for a better nights' sleep (heat exposure affects wakefulness and decreases slow wave sleep and REM sleep . Cold exposure may affect the heart, however. Thus, a cool temperature is best *);

- Make sure you do not set the alarm during a deep sleep phase complete the cycle if you can (cutting the cycle short makes one feel worse on waking; cutting into a light sleep phase is better);
- Get sunlight throughout the day, especially in the morning (this helps to regulate our inner clock and differentiate between day and night);
- Go for a short morning walk to get sunlight and exercise;
- Do not nap longer than 30 minutes and do this earlier in the day;
- Meditate before bed.
- Tighten and relax every muscle, including facial muscles.[38]

And don't forget to affirm for yourself:

I AM LOVED   I AM WELL   I AM GOD'S CHILD

CHAPTER 8:

Exercise

"Since I have been talking to you I see the benefits of exercise; my blood sugar is even better" – Darlene

"Exercise just makes you feel and sleep better'- Diane

"Race walking 3 times a week and I am sleeping good"- Mary

"JUST DO IT" – NIKE

Whether it is going up and down your stairs 10 times a day (not to do laundry, just to exercise), following a YouTube video, jumping rope, jumping jacks, race walking outside, marching in place inside, calisthenics, squats, lunges, burpees, dancing to your favorite music by yourself, JUST DO IT!

Why? How many reasons do you need? Here are a few:

• Boosts the immune system by affecting white blood cells that eliminate bacteria and viruses from the body

- Increases blood flow, and circulation, thus helping to reduce blood pressure
- Reduces stress hormones (adrenaline, which increases your heart rate and blood pressure and cortisol, which increase sugars in the bloodstream – the "fight or flight" hormones) and therefore inflammation
- Increases the body's endorphin levels which are responsible for mood elevation and reducing pain
- Alleviates depression and anxiety
- Increases the level of High Density Lipoproteins (the good cholesterol) and decreases the Low Density Lipoproteins (the bad cholesterol)
- Helps to decreases total cholesterol and triglycerides
- Improves cardiac/ heart function, deterring heart disease, by increasing contractility of heart chambers
- Lowers resting heart rate, and strengthens the heart
- Increases metabolism, or the number of calories you burn a day, which leads to weight loss
- Decreases appetite when you exercise from 20 minute to one hour
- Along with the appropriate food, decreases blood sugar and A1C hemoglobin (the measurement of your blood sugar over a 3 month period of time), and boosts your body's sensitivity to insulin
- insulin sensitivity is increased, and your muscle cells are able to use any available insulin to take up the sugar in your body during exercise and after
- Strengthens bones and strength while toning and firming muscle
- Increases quality of sleep
- Increases self confidence and self esteem when clothes look and feel
- Improves concentration and emotional stability

- Stimulates a feeling of well being and accomplishment

Exercise is a main activity for detoxifying because you are using your lungs exchanging carbon dioxide for oxygen, using the skin by sweating, and if you are drinking more water you are enabling the bladder and the bowels, to eliminate more efficiently.

I have learned to ask patients to start with ten minutes three times a week. When I have asked for more they will say they did not have twenty minutes, for example, so they did nothing. If you have more than ten minutes or can do ten minutes daily, please do so. Start slowly and work up to a race walk if you have not exercised before or are obese. Baby steps are important. You are not preparing for a marathon. And I do want you to set yourself up to win, succeed at whatever goal you set for yourself. At some point I'd like sweating to be a goal.

This past year I have been grieving the death of my mother who lived to be 100. I can tell you, aside from grief counseling, nothing has assisted me more than physical and spiritual exercises, to get through the day.

Do some exercise you love and do it often. Do different exercises. Set goals that you know you can achieve. Maintain a schedule and know this is your time for your self-love and self-care.

You know what to say!

I AM LOVED   I AM WELL   I AM GOD'S CHILD

CHAPTER 9:

Meditation/Spiritual Exercises

"Meditation brings me into a oneness I cannot explain; it quiets the universe, brings comfort, focus and trust. It's centering"
—Diane

"One significant thing you encouraged is meditation; I had worrying thoughts and now they are gone."
—Darlene

A Way To Begin

When I sit down to meditate this is what happens. I say the word "Ani-HU"and then a thought appears. "I have to go to the store," Again I say,"Ani-HU" (said silently breathing out). And another thought

"Call Walter ." "Ani-HU" (breathing out). Another thought. " Remember to send the vitamin D to Ms. Smith," "Ani-HU" (breathing out) " Make the dinner reservation for Sean's birthday", "Ani-HU" (breathing out).

After about 5-10 minutes, I am focused on my breathing and the word "Ani-HU" (I pronounced "an-eye-hue" -I will explain the meaning shortly), and most of the mind chatter is gone.

I have been meditating since 1978, however. Believe me it took time to get to a place of quiet in my mind when I first started. Like many of you, I thought I couldn't do it right or I didn't have the time or the proper altar of incense, or space, or chair, or whatever. In truth, though all of those may make meditation more comfortable, none is essential. Except time.

Just like with exercise you have to take the time. No one is going to give you the time to take care of yourself. It is your responsibility, not anyone else's. Whether your meditation is one minute or one hour, what's important is that you meditate. A patient told me recently she could only sit for a minute. I told her fine! "Sit and focus for one minute, five times a day." During our next visit, she said she was now sitting for five minutes at a time instead of one. This is what I mean by baby steps.

You are not a guru and you will not be able to clear your mind right away. Like anything, learning to meditate takes time and practice. The key is practice. For one to ten minutes each day, I encourage you to sit down and focus on your breathing. You may want to get up after 10 seconds, call your parents, and suddenly do laundry or clean the bathroom. You will have thoughts, and you will think you are doing it wrong. You won't. Just bring your focus and attention back to your breathing. Stay seated. The only wrong way to do it, is not to do it at all.

If you like, you can light a candle and focus on the flame by putting an image of the flame in your mind, preferably between your eyebrows in the location of your pineal gland in the brain. As mentioned in the chapter on sleep, this gland is where melatonin comes from and has an effect on our circadian rhythm. Ancient and current spiritual leaders believe that it is an organ of universal connection that enables our connection to ALL THAT IS, SOURCE or GOD.

You might choose to do an Ayurvedic meditation. Place your two middle fingers on the pulse of your right wrist and feel the pulse for two minutes. It's simple and easy to do. Or try a Tibetan singing bowl meditation where you focus on the sound of the bowls. You can find this meditation on YouTube.

It is not necessary to use the word Ani-HU, and let me tell you why I use it. Hu is a word from Sufism, which is the spiritual aspect of Islam emphasizing the inward search for God. Sufism believes that meditation can bring one closer to God while living and that we do not have to wait until death to experience qualities of or from God. It transcends a particular sect. HU means God. Ani-is a sanskrit (classical language of South Asia/India) word that evokes empathy and compassion for self and others.

Human means God/man. It's a word that denotes the God connection and consciousness in each of us.

I have found that repeating " HU" allows me to go to that place of oneness, compassion, loving, quiet and peace that I can carry throughout my day. That place that enables me to listen, focus and fulfill my purpose here, day to day, by giving me the inner connection to the Source of all things. Meditation brings me into the present moment. There is no past and future there is only now. And when I find myself not in "now", it is easier to get back to "now" because of my meditation practice. During and after my meditation I experience an energy that is sweet, still, Grace-filled, peaceful, forgiving and compassionate. I recognize there is a place inside of me that is one with All That Is. That place that loves all, forgives all, has compassion for all and gratitude for the oneness. Meditation allows for being in the present moment, listening. Ideas and awareness come as well during, and after meditation.

Prayer is talking to God. Meditation is listening to God. I have heard patients say that their pastors warned them against meditating, calling it anti religious or even worse, blasphemous. Meditation is non-denominational.

It is not a religion or a philosophy or even a way of being, rather it's meditating on the Light within you. Every religion teaches that having a God consciousness and having a personal relationship with God is essential for well-being. For me, that has been, and continues to be true. And God is in all things, everywhere, all the time, including you and me.

We are made in the image of Mother/Father God.

I am not a biblical scholar, however, I am aware of this Bible verse: "And the Word was made flesh, and dwelt among us, full of grace and truth" (John 1:14 KJV). Of course, it is speaking of Jesus Christ, who was God and human. We are all His brothers and sisters, children of God. I believe He came to show us the way to be loving and forgiving of ourselves and others. I believe we are all a part of God and our flesh is the temple where we can go to seek God and experience forgiveness and lovingkindness. Similarly, the Bible says "Seek ye first the kingdom of heaven (God) and all else will be added unto you" (Matthew 6:33). And in the New King James version in Luke 17:20-21 it says " The Kingdom of God will not come with observable signs. Nor will people say, 'See here', or 'See there' it is. For indeed the kingdom of God is within you."

All day I hear my patients talk about the anxiety, depression, fear, and anger they feel because of all that's going on in the world. Those things only add to the day-to-day stresses of family, children, work, relationships, and economic concerns. Meditation is not a panacea, but it is a way to reduce the cascading of stress hormones that begin whenever we hear the news (whether from a friend or TV) of racial discrimination, police brutality, or civil unrest.

The Effects of Meditation

Many of us live with chronic stress. Whether it is about not being able to pay your bills or worrying about having "the conversation" with your son, nephew, or younger brother about what to do when pulled over by the police, the constant pumping of cortisol and adrenaline throughout our bodies affects our genes and increases our predisposition for high blood pressure, diabetes, heart disease, obesity, and cancer— not to mention the damage it does to our mental health.

Stress may be a boss or co-worker who is demeaning and rude. Or the news that is negative and threatening, a friend who is jealous or one who is depressed and anxious, a child on drugs, a parent or sibling with dementia, an ex-partner or current one, your grief, or a simple deadline at work. That mixed with the pressures to keep up on social media, creates constant stress. We need to have something in our lives to stop this bombardment, even if for a moment. We need to have something in our lives to stop the energy of anger, guilt, and resentment, that has become part of our daily existence. This energy makes us sick. We must focus on our inner world and let the outer world stop influencing us, again, even for a moment. This is about breaking old habits of thought, feeling and doing and creating new ones so that you can create a new you in every moment. Those old habits take us out of the present and keep us tied to the past. If there is an event about which you are angry, write about it, without proper English and use curse words if that pleases you, and burn it. Do this as many times as you need to release negative thoughts and feelings from your past.

I learned early on in a seminar called Insight, that energy is just that, energy. We decide how to use it. For example, anxiety and excitement are both energies. You cannot touch those emotions. Pretend you have a coin to go into a juke box and you can pick any song you like. Anxiety and excitement are the same energy. You can choose anxiety about the job interview or excitement about the job interview. Through meditation, the energy of anxiety will be less familiar to you and therefore will not be the first emotion you choose anymore. You will become aware of options. As with homeopathy, the remedy, which is energy, gets rid of the energy that the body has created in response to some event, thus changing the electromagnetic field (of the immune system) of the person. Unworthiness to increased self- esteem, rage to peace, anxiety to calm, and guilt to forgiveness are all possible with meditation as well.

Meditation then can stop so much emotional eating of the comfort food that can be responsible for the dis-eases we experience disproportionately. " Stress affects the same signals as famine does. It turns on the brain pathways that make us crave dense calories—we'll choose high fat, high sweet foods or high salt," says Dr. Elissa Epel, the founder of Center for Obesity Assessment, Study and Treatment at the University of California San Francisco.* By calming the central nervous system and our emotions, we are able to have more control over what we eat, when we eat and how much we eat.[39]

Essentially, meditation reduces stress and the releasing of stress hormones like cytokines which create inflammation. Meditation also decreases the risk of heart disease, increases our concentration and attention span, can improve our sleep patterns, help control pain, increases self-awareness, and promote compassion and positive thinking.

There are many ways to meditate. Choose one and try it for thirty days. If you miss a day please do not beat yourself up. Just like when a patient misses a day during the detoxification diet, I tell them to go to the next meal and make it even healthier. Similarly, with meditation, we are detoxifying our spirit. Whatever you do, do not judge yourself, just go to the next day and discover what is inside.

I AM LOVED   I AM WELL   I AM GOD'S CHILD

SALVATION

The Act Of Protecting From Harm, Risk, Loss;
Preservation Or Deliverance From Harm, Risk, Loss;
The State Of Being Protected
From A Dire Situation.

CHAPTER 10:

The Truth As I Know It

It doesn't matter where you are in your process toward having a healthier life or how you got where you are. Wherever you are, you can change. Creating good health is not linear and does not happen overnight. None of my Superwomen became suddenly healthy and happy. It took time to change their old habits. The key is they could see the value of the incremental changes, and that encouraged them to stay focused and keep going.

I believe in life it is helpful to have a vision. And if you are going to have a vision, have a big vision. In addition to treating your hypertension or diabetes, who, what and how do you want to be in the world? How do you want to live? How do you want to feel? What do you want to look like in two to five years? Decide you are going to change and how you want to change. Write it out. What is your intention? Having an intention makes the methods to get there show up.

Many years ago, I learned in a seminar called Insight how to create a vision board, and I created the life I wanted on that board. I cut out pictures and statements from magazines of the life I wanted and taped them on the poster board. I have pictures of Serena Williams with the words " love your body", Oprah with the words " more than enough" and words "experience amazing" and "living well" on the board. There are names and pictures of countries where I wanted to travel as well. It was fun doing it and it has been fascinating to see how much of my life is on the board. There were disappointments – a failed marriage, and another that never happened and financial setbacks during the 2008 market – for sure.

But I never stopped faithing, believing, growing, learning and seeking, and God made a way out of no way. With each set-back I picked myself up, and I learned that setbacks were God's way of pruning me so I could dig my roots deeper, reach my limbs higher and experience greater self love, self-confidence and a stronger faith in God.

Self-love is a must, it's non-negotiable, but if you don't already have it, you won't cultivate it overnight. That's okay, because the more you do for yourself the more love you have for yourself, and the more love you have for yourself, the more you do for yourself. So, start doing for yourself! Remember, self-love is not dependent on how others treat you. It is about how you treat you. It doesn't matter what your parents or relatives said or didn't say about you. Forgive them and move on. You must do whatever is necessary to get rid of beliefs that hold you back. Start by telling yourself you love yourself. State this while looking at yourself in the mirror, every day, until you believe it. Also write it out. Also say it as you wrap your arms around yourself in a big warm hug.

Sometimes, self-love means disconnecting from people who do not have your best interest in mind. Those people could be family members or friends. Read, go online and listen to self-improvement podcasts

(YouTube, Yale University, Science of Being Well, Insight, Seminars, Achieve Today). Depending on how much trauma you've experienced, you may benefit from therapy and of course homeopathy. Seeking therapy doesn't mean you are crazy. It means you have been living in America as an African- American woman with a cultural history of slavery and all of its chains. It means you have come this far doing what you do, and it has gotten you where you are. Be grateful and list those blessings. You have survived and persevered. If you are happy where you are, fine. If not, make the decision to take charge of your life and dare to thrive.

Still, take baby steps. Every day do something to change your life. It can be anything from getting up fifteen minutes earlier to simply moving your body for fifteen minutes or drinking water before breakfast. An accountability partner always helps. Ask a neighbor or relative or a friend to hold you accountable for whatever goals you've committed to.

It is true you manifest what you believe, and the universe is here to support you. List your blessings, focus on them and be grateful now. Don't wait until you get that degree or job or start your business or write a book. Be grateful now. Act as if it has already happened. God loves and supports you and God has to know what you want. You have to meet God halfway by moving in the direction of what you say you want. I tell my patients all the time, if you want to buy a car you have to go online or go to the car lot. The car is not going to come crashing through your living room window.

God did not intend for you to be ill and upset and depressed all the time. God did not put you here in this thing called life to dump you and never assist you. Life is precious and so are you. Please take care of yourself. The planet needs you. Do something daily that gives you strength spiritually, mentally, emotionally and physically.

One of the participants in the documentary "The Secret", Bob Doyle, stated simply "create a new life from scratch." Below I share more of the Truth as I know it:

- Realize you are more than enough.
- Be responsible for what you put in your, body, mind and soul. You are the temple where God resides.
- Take time to go inside and explore. There is so much outside yourself that distracts you and gives you false messages. Go inside.
- No one is responsible for your joy or lack thereof. That is between you and your God. The kingdom of heaven is within. Go there.
- How can you have more peace? Stop being at war with yourself and others.
- Laugh more today than yesterday.
- Thoughts are powerful and negative thoughts in particular are addictive, habitual and stressful. Start having positive thoughts.
- Forgive yourself for judging yourself and others as wrong.
- Be faithful. It is easy to be faithful when things are going great. Faith is believing that things are perfect even when they are not great.
- Everything is perfect, especially when you do not like it.
- Acceptance is the first law of Spirit – accept all of you and commit to change.
- Are you a Superwoman? There always is and always will be something to do for someone else. Do something for you today.
- As Serena Williams says, "Never Give up."
- As Mary Lou Sullivan said, "Know that everything is going to be alright."

I AM LOVED   I AM WELL   I AM GOD'S CHILD

Epilogue

Bring What Has Worked For You Into The Now And Move Forward:

F = Faithing, Forgiveness

O = Organic – Natural Life Or Living Matter

R = Renew Self, Reward Self, Recreate Self Through Daily Ritual

W = Water, Winner, Wisdom (Inner)

A = Ask For What You Want, Affirmation

R = Rejoice/Give Thanks

D = Divinity/God's Child

And Celebrate:

C = Choice, Create Your Life Day To Day Moment To Moment

E = Empower Yourself

L = Love Yourself

E = Easy – Be Gentle With Yourself

B = Be Brave And Bold

R = Rest And Rejuvenate

A = Acceptance

T = Tell Your Truth

E = Energy Is Available To You When Making Life Changes

We are super women. We are bold, bright, beautiful, daring, caring, charitable, creative, nurturing, faithful, strong, delicate, fearless, powerful, sensitive, loving, kind, formidable, vulnerable and gracious. Let us be a part of the cycle of giving and receiving to and from ourselves, such that we know WELLNESS is but one more example of God's Grace.

God bless us all.

Biography

Dr. Sullivan received an ND (Doctor of Naturopathic Medicine) degree from Bastyr University in Seattle, Washington in 1986. After graduating from the four year accredited program, Dr. Sullivan also took advanced courses in Homeopathic medicine in the United States, India and Europe. She continues to study with Homeopathic physicians from Mumbai (Bombay) India and is a diplomat with the Homeopathic Academy of Naturopathic Physicians. She has a private practice in Washington, D.C.

In 1976, Dr. Sullivan was the first African American to receive a PhD from the University of Pennsylvania in Sociology/Criminology. She taught at Howard University, American University and the University of Maryland, and was subsequently appointed Assistant Director of the Administration of Justice for the National Urban League in New York City. She later worked as a special assistant for urban policy to Patricia Roberts Harris, the U.S Secretary of Housing and Urban Development (HUD) during the Carter administration.

Dr. Sullivan is a founding member of the American Association of Naturopathic Physicians and served as president of the D.C. Association of Naturopathic Physicians for eight years. In 2007, she was also appointed by the mayor of the nation's capital to serve as chairperson of the Naturopathic Medical Board for the District of Columbia, after having served on the Board of Medicine for 5 years.

Excerpts from her successful first book, A Path to Healing: A Guide to Wellness for Body, Mind, and Soul (April 1998; Doubleday), appeared in Essence Magazine in July 1998, followed by several feature stories on Dr. Sullivan over the following years. Dr. Sullivan is also a contributing writer to Prevention, Essence, Ebony, Huffington Post Heart and Soul and Health Quest publications. She has also a presentations/ discussions on YouTube.

Her second book, tentatively entitled, Enough: When Sacrifice Has Gone Too Far, will be released in 2021.

She is also featured in the 2013 African American History Calendar for Aetna Health Insurance.

Dr. Sullivan is frequently a guest on radio and major network television, and travels throughout the country and Canada to lecture on Naturopathic medicine and wellness.[40]

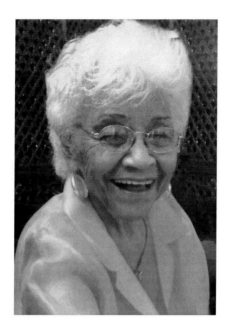

This book is dedicated to the memory of my mother

Mary Lucretia Harris Sullivan

August 22, 1919 - September 24, 2019

Index

References

1 Mullings, L. (2002). The Sojourner Syndrome: Race, Class, and Gender in Health and Illness. Voices, 6(1), 32-36. doi:10.1525/vo.2002.6.1.3

2 Craig, Maxine Leeds, Ain't I A Beauty Queen: Black Women, Beauty and the Politics of Race, Oxford University Press USA, 2002 p. 7).

3 Winkler, Karen J. The Life of the Legendary Sojourner Truth: A New Biography Explores The Facts and Fictions, The Chronicle of Higher Education 43.3;

4 US History .org, National Historical Park Women's Rights Quaker Influence

5 Atlas Obscura March 27, 2017. The 1920's Women Who Fougt For The Right To Travel Under Their Own Names.

6 Woods-Giscombé CL. Superwoman schema: African American women's views on stress, strength, and health. Qual Health Res. 2010;20(5):668-683. doi:10.1177/1049732310361892

7 Ostchega Y, Fryar CD, Nwankwo T, Nguyen DT. Hypertension Prevalence Among Adults Aged 18 and Over: United States, 2017-2018. NCHS Data Brief. 2020 Apr;(364):1-8. PMID: 3248729

8 Richardson LC, Henley SJ, Miller JW, Massetti G, Thomas CC. Patterns and Trends in Age-Specific Black-White Differences in Breast Cancer Incidence and Mortality – United States, 1999–2014. MMWR Morb Mortal Wkly Rep 2016;65:1093–1098. DOI: http://dx.doi.org/10.15585/mmwr.mm6540a1

9 "Office of Minority Health." Diabetes and African Americans - The Office of Minority Health, minorityhealth.hhs.gov/omh/browse.aspx?lvl=4&lvlid=18.

10 Banister CE, Messersmith AR, Cai B, et al. Disparity in the persistence of high-risk human papillomavirus genotypes between African American and European American women of college age. J Infect Dis. 2015;211(1):100-108. doi:10.1093/infdis/jiu394

11 Kimball, R. (2020). Who rules?: Sovereignty, nationalism, and the fate of freedom in the twenty-first century. NY, NY: Encounter Books.

12 Williams RA. Cardiovascular disease in African American women: a health care disparities issue. J Natl Med Assoc. 2009 Jun;101(6):536-40. doi: 10.1016/s0027-9684(15)30938-x. PMID: 19585921.

13 Holly Corbett, " Why Black women's equal payday is so important", Forbes, August 13, 2020

14 US Bureau of Labor Statistics: Labor Force Statistics from the Current Population Survey. E-16 Unemployment rates by age , sex, race, and Hispanic or Latino Ethnicity. January 2021. www.bls.gov/ CPS

15 Bieiweis,B., Boesch,D, and Cawthorne Gaines,A. August 3, 2020Center for American Progress , The Basic Facts About Women in Poverty

16 Villarosa, Linda. Body & Soul: the Black Womens Guide to Physical Health and Emotional Well-Being. Vermilion, 2003.

17 Black and White. (n.d.). Retrieved from https://www. nationalgeographic.com/magazine/issue/april-2018

18 The Race Issue, National Geographic,, March 2018, p. 31

19 Mitchell, P. W. (n.d.). The fault in his seeds: Lost notes to the case of bias in Samuel George Morton's cranial race science. Retrieved from https://journals.plos.org/plosbiology/article?id=10.1371/journal. pbio.2007008

20 Black and White. (n.d.). Retrieved from https://www. nationalgeographic.com/magazine/issue/april-2018

21 Lust, Benedict. Naturopath and Herald of Health. Benedict Lust, 1937.

22 J;, A. R. (n.d.). Plain water consumption in relation to energy intake and diet quality among US adults, 2005-2012. Retrieved from https://pubmed.ncbi.nlm.nih.gov/26899737/

23 Popkin, B. M., Danci, K. E., & Rosenberg, I. H. (2010). Water, hydration, and health. Nutrition Reviews, 68(8), 439-458. doi:10.1111/j.1753-4887.2010.00304.x

24 DiNicolantonio JJ, O'Keefe JH, Wilson WLSugar addiction: is it real? A narrative reviewBritish Journal of Sports Medicine 2018;52:910-913.

25 Yang Q, Zhang Z, Gregg EW, Flanders WD, Merritt R, Hu FB. Added sugar intake and cardiovascular diseases mortality among US adults. JAMA Intern Med. 2014 Apr;174(4):516-24. doi: 10.1001/jamainternmed.2013.13563. PMID: 24493081.

26 Weber KS, Simon MC, Strassburger K, Markgraf DF, Buyken AE, Szendroedi J, Müssig K, Roden M; GDS Group. Habitual Fructose Intake Relates to Insulin Sensitivity and Fatty Liver Index in Recent-Onset Type 2 Diabetes Patients and Individuals without Diabetes. Nutrients. 2018 Jun 15;10(6):774. doi: 10.3390/nu10060774. PMID: 29914103; PMCID: PMC6024554.

27 Dornas WC, de Lima WG, Pedrosa ML, Silva ME. Health implications of high-fructose intake and current research. Adv Nutr. 2015;6(6):729-737. Published 2015 Nov 13. doi:10.3945/an.114.008144

28 Anton SD, Martin CK, Han H, Coulon S, Cefalu WT, Geiselman P, Williamson DA. Effects of stevia, aspartame, and sucrose on food intake, satiety, and postprandial glucose and insulin levels. Appetite.

2010 Aug;55(1):37-43. doi: 10.1016/j.appet.2010.03.009. Epub 2010 Mar 18. PMID: 20303371; PMCID: PMC2900484.

29 Ahmad U, Ahmad RS, Arshad MS, Mushtaq Z, Hussain SM, Hameed A. Antihyperlipidemic efficacy of aqueous extract of Stevia rebaudiana Bertoni in albino rats. Lipids Health Dis. 2018 Jul 27;17(1):175. doi: 10.1186/s12944-018-0810-9. PMID: 30053819; PMCID: PMC6064095.

30 Aune D, Navarro Rosenblatt DA, Chan DS, Vieira AR, Vieira R, Greenwood DC, Vatten LJ, Norat T. Dairy products, calcium, and prostate cancer risk: a systematic review and meta-analysis of cohort studies. Am J Clin Nutr. 2015 Jan;101(1):87-117. doi: 10.3945/ajcn.113.067157. Epub 2014 Nov 19. PMID: 25527754.

31 DiNicolantonio JJ, O'Keefe JH, Wilson WLSugar addiction: is it real? A narrative reviewBritish Journal of Sports Medicine 2018;52:910-913.

32 Dahl-Jørgensen K, Joner G, Hanssen KF. Relationship between cows' milk consumption and incidence of IDDM in childhood. Diabetes Care. 1991 Nov;14(11):1081-3. doi: 10.2337/diacare.14.11.1081. PMID: 1797491.

33 Malosse D, Perron H, Sasco A, Seigneurin JM. Correlation between milk and dairy product consumption and multiple sclerosis prevalence: a worldwide study. Neuroepidemiology. 1992;11(4-6):304-12. doi: 10.1159/000110946. PMID: 1291895.

34 Rona RJ, Keil T, Summers C, Gislason D, Zuidmeer L, Sodergren E, Sigurdardottir ST, Lindner T, Goldhahn K, Dahlstrom J, McBride D, Madsen C. The prevalence of food allergy: a meta-analysis. J Allergy